Occupational Therapy and Stroke

Occupational Therapy and Stroke

Edited by

JUDI EDMANS, ANNETTE CHAMPION, LOUISE HILL, MIKE RIDLEY, FIONA SKELLY, THERESE JACKSON & MOYA NEALE

Stroke Clinical Forum of the National Association of Neurological Occupational Therapists (NANOT)

Consulting Editor in Occupational Therapy
CLEPHANE HUME

W

WHURR PUBLISHERS
LONDON AND PHILADELPHIA

© 2001 Whurr Publishers
First published 2001 by
Whurr Publishers Ltd
19b Compton Terrace, London N1 2UN, England and
325 Chestnut Street, Philadelphia PA 19106, USA

Reprinted 2001 (twice), 2002, 2003 and 2005

British Library Cataloguing in Publication Data
A catalogue record for this book is available from the
British Library.

ISBN: 186156 198 9

Printed and bound in the UK by Athenaeum Press Ltd,
Gateshead, Tyne & Wear

Contents

Preface

This book has been produced by the stroke clinical forum members of the National Association of Neurological Occupational Therapists (NANOT) (UK), which is a specialist section of the College of Occupational Therapists. The book is intended for use by newly qualified occupational therapists and those new to the field of stroke management. It acknowledges the many different techniques that may be used in stroke management and the scope of the occupational therapy role in the UK. We have tried to offer a guide through the maze of problems that present in stroke patients, with suggestions for their management. We hope that, by providing guidance, new graduates will feel confident in their management of stroke patients.

Chapters are presented in a form that enables the therapist to review the subject prior to assessment and treatment planning. Complex problems are grouped together to avoid confusion. We hope this book will encourage therapists to use their skills in observation and problem solving, adapting and building on the techniques seen on clinical placement and taught in college.

Stroke continues to be a major condition seen by occupational therapists in both hospitals and the community. The book enables the therapist to apply the rehabilitation principles wherever he/she encounters stroke patients, i.e. in hospital or community and whatever their age or culture.

National government policies in the UK now require therapy be supported by evidence of effectiveness. The section on evaluation helps the therapist monitor standards of intervention and its effectiveness.

Throughout this book the patient/client is referred to as 'the patient', for ease of terminology, irrespective of whether he/she is being treated in hospital or in the community.

Thanks are extended to everyone who has assisted in the production of this book. Particular thanks go to Judi Edmans, who has kept everyone on target to reach our deadlines; and to Moya Neale and Fiona Skelly, who have both chaired the working group.

Finally, in the future, as new ideas are developed, this text should be viewed in the light of developing practice.

Annette Champion
NANOT Chairman 1995–98

Stroke: Good Practice in Occupational Therapy

The government White Paper produced in 1998, *A First Class Service*, placed quality at the top of the NHS agenda, setting out a package of measures to promote quality and reduce variations in service provision. National mechanisms include the National Institute of Clinical Excellence (NICE), National Service Frameworks (NSF), Commission for Health Improvement (CHImp), National Performance Framework and the National Survey of Patient and User Experience.

NSFs will set national standards and produce service models for a defined group or care group. They will also put in place strategies to support implementations and establish performance measures against which progress within an agreed time-scale can be measured.

The National Service Framework for older people is supported by several task groups, one of which has the responsibility for stroke. This group aims to produce minimum recommended standards of care for stroke patients across the country and I represented NANOT/COT on this group. Evidence-based practice is recommended and we have referred to the Royal College of Physicians' National Clinical Guidelines for Stroke. The standards will cover health promotion and stroke prevention, immediate management, rehabilitation in both hospital and the community, and longer-term support. At NANOT, in line with government initiatives, we are promoting the development of Occupational Therapy specific standards for people with stroke and this book goes a long way to provide the foundations for good practice.

Therese Jackson
NANOT Chairman 1998–2000

Patient/Staff Ratio

For the acute/intensive rehabilitation of patients following stroke, a ratio of one occupational therapist to five patients is recommended by the National Association of Neurological Occupational Therapists.

List of Contributors

Thanks go to all the following people, who have contributed to the production of this stroke resource pack:

- Tina Ashburner, Stoke Mandeville Hospital, Aylesbury
- Sarah Broughton, The Wellington Hospital, London
- Annette Champion, Community Neuro Rehabilitation Team, Croydon
- Emma Charles, Ayrshire Hospital, Ayrshire
- Colleen Cherry, Royal Hallamshire Hospital, Sheffield
- Patricia Church, Queens Medical Centre, Nottingham
- Moira Conion-Scott, South Tyneside District Hospital, South Shields.
- Richard Davies, Sheffield Hallam University
- Avril Drummond, Queens Medical Centre, Nottingham
- Judi Edmans, City Hospital, Nottingham
- Louise Hill, West Herts Rehabilitation Service, Watford
- Therese Jackson, King's College Hospital, London
- Chris Murray, Queen's Medical Centre, Nottingham
- Moya Neale, Bronglais Hospital, Aberystwyth
- Mike Ridley, South Tyneside District Hospital, South Shields
- Christine Sealey, College of Occupational Therapists, London
- Fiona Skelly, Firth Park Clinic, Sheffield
- Penny Spreadbury, City Hospital, Nottingham
- Eleanor Stout, City Hospital, Nottingham
- Sue Vernon, Banstead Mobility Centre, Carshalton
- Marion Walker, City Hospital, Nottingham

Chapter 1
Introduction

Definition of Stroke (Aho et al., 1980)

The World Health Organisation (WHO) defines stroke as 'rapidly developed clinical signs of focal (or global) disturbances of cerebral function, lasting more than 24 hours or leading to death, with no apparent cause other than vascular origin'.

Causes of Stroke

The main causes of stroke are:

1. *Ischaemia leading to infarction* (i.e. deficient blood supply leading to area of tissue deprived of blood supply usually caused by an embolism from heart, aorta, carotid or vertebral vessels):
   - *embolus* (obstruction, e.g. by blood clot, fat, tumour or air bubble moving);
   - *thrombus* (stationary blood clot formed in cerebral artery);
   - *lacunae* (tiny infarcts located deeply within brain);
   - *hypoperfusion/microemboli* (infarct in area between two major arterial territories, 'watershed');
   - *TIA* (transient ischaemic attack, lasting less than 24 hours).
2. *Haemorrhage* (i.e. escape of blood from a vessel caused by hypertension or abnormal clotting. This could be in *subarachnoid, subdural, intracerebral* or *extradural* areas):
   - *aneurysm* (bulge in weak artery wall);
   - *arterio-venous malformation* (malformation of the arterio-venous structure);
   - *trauma* (RTA/head injury).

Classification of Stroke

Bamford (1991) described a classification of cerebral infarction, to aid clinicians in identifying groups of patients with similar deficits. This classification is based on the signs exhibited and symptoms experienced by patients.

This classification was as follows:

- *Total Anterior Circulation Infarction* (TACI):
    - motor and sensory deficit, ipsilateral hemianopia and new distur
      bance of higher cerebral function;
- *Partial Anterior Circulation Infarction* (PACI):
    - any two of the above; or
    - isolated disturbance of higher cerebral function;
- *Posterior Circulation Infarction* (POCI):
    - unequivocal signs of brainstem disturbance; or
    - isolated hemianopia;
- *Lacunar Infarction* (LACI):
    - pure motor stroke; or
    - pure sensory stroke; or
    - pure sensorimotor stroke; or
    - ataxic hemiparesis.

International Classification of Impairments, Disabilities and Handicaps (WHO, Aho et al., 1980)

The World Health Organisation described the following classification:

- *Pathology*: damaged processes within an organ or system in the body, e.g. *stroke*;
- *Impairment*: disordered function due to pathology, signs and symptoms, e.g. *ataxia, unable to move upper or lower limb*;
- *Disability*: loss of functional ability due to pathology or impairment, e.g. *unable to dress or walk*;
- *Handicap:* social disadvantage due to impairment or disability, e.g. *unable to live at home independently*.

This model is currently being revised by the WHO (Badley, 1997) as it uses negative terminology. The new terms will be *pathology, impairment, activity* and *participation*:

- *Pathology*: damaged processes within an organ or system in the body, e.g. *stroke*;
- *Impairment*: loss or abnormality of body structure or of physiological or psychological function;
- *Activity*: (replacing disability) nature and extent of functioning and activity limitations;
- *Participation*: (replacing handicap) involvement in life situations or restrictions experienced in participation in life situations.

Medical Investigations of Patients Following Stroke or Transient Ischaemic Attack

After suffering a stroke or transient ischaemic attack (TIA), a number of investigations are often performed. The aims of these investigations are:

- to confirm the diagnosis of stroke;
- to determine the site and pathology of the stroke;
- to establish the cause(s) of the stroke;
- to prevent further strokes.

Computerised Tomography (CT) or Magnetic Resonance Imaging (MRI)

This helps establish the pathological diagnosis by showing cerebral infarction or haemorrhage and excluding other conditions that may mimic stroke (tumours, subdural haematomas, etc.). The distinction between haemorrhage and infarction is important as treatment with aspirin or anticoagulants is likely to be indicated for cerebral infarction but would be contraindicated in cerebral haemorrhage. A CT scan should therefore be performed in all patients in whom active treatment is considered.

It is difficult to distinguish haemorrhage from infarction on CT if the patient is scanned after about two weeks. MRI is more useful in this situation. It is also better at demonstrating small infarcts and lesions in the brainstem and cerebellum.

Stroke patients often have a normal CT if they are scanned within the first few hours after stroke. The CT will become abnormal if repeated after a few days, but there are still some patients who have a definite stroke despite normal CT scans.

Blood Tests

- *Full blood count*: to look for conditions that predispose to clotting such as polycythaemia (increased red cells), thrombocythaemia (increased platelets) and conditions that predispose to haemorrhage, e.g. thrombocytopenia (decreased platelets);
- *Erythrocyte sedimentation rate* (ESR): if raised suggests infection, vasculitis or carcinoma and should lead to further investigation;
- *Blood sugar*: is essential to exclude diabetes mellitus;
- *Fasting lipids*: are checked in all but the very elderly so that appropriate lipid-lowering strategies can be started;
- *Clotting screen*: an investigation of blood clotting is needed in patients with haemorrhagic stroke;
- *Thrombophilia screen*: young patients with ischaemic stroke or transient ischaemic attack (TIA) need special blood tests to look for rare causes of

thrombophilia, e.g. protein C&S, antithrombin III, and anticardiolipin autoantibodies;
- *Syphilis serology*: neurosyphilis is still a rare cause of stroke and TIA, and needs to be specifically looked for in most patients;
- *Blood cultures*: if endocarditis is suspected.

Cardiac Investigations

There is a cardiac source of embolism in 30% of cases of cerebral infarction.

- *ECG*: should be performed in all patients looking for atrial fibrillation and any evidence of myocardial damage;
- *Echocardiogram*: is performed in selected patients (especially the young) to identify any potential cardiac source of emboli.

Carotid Ultrasound

This is performed to identify internal carotid artery stenosis, occlusion and dissection. Emboli from this artery are responsible for about 10% of ischaemic strokes. The technique involves imaging of the artery with measurement of blood-flow velocity, which allows an estimation of the degree of vessel stenosis to be made.

Catheter Digital Subtraction Angiography

This is a sophisticated investigation involving the direct injection of contrast into arteries. It carries a 1% risk of stroke. It is used to confirm carotid stenosis (after ultrasound) prior to carotid surgery, to diagnose the source of bleeding in patients with haemorrhagic stroke, and occasionally in patients with unexplained symptoms.

Magnetic Resonance Angiography

This is beginning to provide an alternative technique for imaging the carotid and vertebral arteries. It is non-invasive and involves assimilating cross-sectional MR scans to provide images of the arteries. Where available, this technique will allow more patients to be investigated without the need for catheter angiography.

Prevention of Recurrence of Stroke (Secondary Prevention)

After an individual suffers a stroke, many strategies are used to help prevent recurrence. General measures are recommended in all patients, such as reducing weight, stopping smoking and taking regular exercise.

Aspirin

After ischaemic stroke or TIA, aspirin reduces the risk of further vascular events by 20%. The optimal dosage is not known, but probably 300 mg daily is a reasonable starting dose and can be reduced if there are side effects. Dipyridamole (Persantin) is sometimes used if there is intolerance to aspirin. There are newer antiplatelet drugs now developed such as ticlopidine and clopidrogel but these are expensive and not in common usage in the UK.

Blood Pressure and Diabetes

Hypertension is the single most important risk factor for stroke and should be actively treated in all hypertensive patients. Likewise diabetic control must also be optimal following a stroke.

Hyperlipidaemia

This should be treated with diet or drugs. There is no good evidence that treatment reduces stroke risk but there is evidence that death from coronary artery disease is reduced.

Anticoagulants

There are many conditions in which treatment with Warfarin reduces the risk of stroke. Clinical trials have demonstrated the benefit of Warfarin in the prevention of stroke in patients with atrial fibrillation. Warfarin is also indicated for patients with valvular heart disease, other suspected cardiac sources of embolism, prothrombotic states (e.g. protein C&S deficiency) and for recurrent TIAs or stroke with no obvious cause.

There is a risk of haemorrhage for patients taking Warfarin, and therefore it is not indicated in patients who have a predisposition to haemorrhage (e.g. peptic ulcers), or in patients who would have difficulty complying accurately with medication. Aspirin is an alternative in some patients for whom Warfarin would not be suitable.

Carotid Endarterectomy

Trials have shown that this operation to widen the internal carotid artery is highly beneficial in preventing stroke in symptomatic patients with recent TIA or stroke. It is useful only in patients with a severe stenosis (>70%) and should be limited to reasonably fit patients under 85 years of age. St George's Hospital, London, is currently coordinating a large trial of angioplasty (widening the artery with a balloon) of the internal carotid and vertebral arteries. This technique in principle has many advantages over conventional surgery (no anaesthetic, much shorter time in hospital) but cannot be widely recommended until the results of trials are available.

Preventive Neurosurgery

Patients who have suffered from haemorrhagic stroke (primary intracerebral haemorrhage, subarachnoid haemorrhage) often have an underlying arterial abnormality such as an aneurysm or arterio-venous malformation. Further haemorrhage from these sites can often be prevented by neurosurgical techniques such as aneurysm clipping or embolization of A-V malformations.

Damage That Can Occur in Different Areas of the Brain

Testani-Dufour and Marano Morrison (1997) described the arterial supply of the brain and the results of occlusion of those arteries. They also described the functions of the different areas of the brain and the deficits that can occur as a result of damage to those areas. This information is collated in Tables 1.1–1.3.

Table 1.1 Anterior circulation

Ophthalmic artery

Supplies
- orbit
- optic nerve

Occlusion
- transient mononuclear blindness (amaurosis fugax)
- complete unilateral blindness

Anterior choroidal artery

Supplies
- deep structures of the brain (basal ganglia, thalamus, posterior limb of internal capsule and medial temporal lobe)

Occlusion
- contralateral hemiplegia, hemihypesthesia, homonymous hemianopia

Anterior cerebral artery

Supplies
- anterior 3/4 of medial surface of cerebral hemisphere
- portions of the basal ganglia
- internal capsule

Occlusion
- contralateral sensory and motor deficits foot and leg > arm
- face and hand not usually involved
- incontinence
- deviation of eyes and head towards lesion
- contralateral grasp reflex
- abulic symptoms (apathy, decreased spontaneity, limited speech)

Left ACA
- arm apraxia
- expressive aphasia

Distal ACA
- contralateral upper and lower extremity weakness
- contralateral sensory loss in foot
- motor and/or sensory aphasia

Table 1.1 contd.

Middle cerebral artery

Supplies
- basal ganglia
- fibres of internal capsule
- cortical surfaces of the parietal, temporal and frontal lobes

Complete occlusion
- contralateral gaze palsy
- hemiplegia
- hemisensory loss
- spatial neglect
- homonymous hemianopia
- global aphasia (with left hemisphere lesions)

Occlusion superior trunk of MCA
- contralateral hemiplegia
- hemianaesthesia in face and arm > leg
- ipsilateral deviation eyes and head
- Broca's aphasia (with dominant hemisphere lesion)

Occlusion inferior trunk of MCA
- contralateral hemianopia or upper quadrantopia
- Wernicke's aphasia (usually with left-sided lesions)
- left visual neglect (usually with right-sided lesions)
- motor or sensory deficit usually absent

Table 1.2 Posterior circulation

Vertebral artery

Supplies
- anterolateral parts of the medulla

Occlusion
(lateral medullary syndrome)
- contralateral impairment pain and temperature sensation
- ipsilateral Horner's syndrome
- dysphagia
- decreased gag reflex
- vertigo
- nystagmus
- ataxia

Table 1.2 contd.

Posterior inferior cerebellar artery

Supplies
- medulla
- cerebellum

Occlusion medial branch
- vertigo
- nystagmus
- ataxia
- persistent dizziness

Occlusion lateral branch
- unilateral clumsiness
- gait and limb ataxia
- inability to stand or sudden fall often
- vertigo
- dysarthria
- nystagmus
- eye deviation

Basilar artery

Supplies
- pons
- midbrain

Occlusion
- limb paralysis
- bulbar or pseudobulbar paralysis of the cranial nerve motor nuclei
- nystagmus
- eye movement disturbance
- coma

Complete occlusion
- locked in syndrome
- consciousness with complete motor paralysis, inability to communicate orally or by gesture

Posterior choroidal artery

Supplies
- third ventricle
- dorsal surface of thalamus

Occlusion
- not seen

Posterior cerebral artery

Supplies
- occipital lobe
- medial and inferior surface of temporal lobe
- midbrain
- third and lateral ventricles

Occlusion
- contralateral hemiplegia
- sensory loss
- ipsilateral visual field deficits
- weakness greater in face and upper extremities

Table 1.2 contd.

Anterior inferior cerebellar artery

Supplies
- cerebellum
- pons

Occlusion
- vertigo
- nausea
- vomiting
- nystagmus
- tinnitus
- ipsilateral cerebellar ataxia
- Horner's syndrome
- contralateral loss of pain and temperature sense of arm, trunk and leg

Superior cerebellar artery

Supplies
- cerebellum upper part
- midbrain

Occlusion
- ipsilateral cerebellar ataxia
- nausea
- vomiting
- slurred speech
- contralateral loss of pain and thermal sensation

Table 1.3 Areas of the brain

Frontal lobe

Functions
- concentration
- abstract thought
- memory
- judgement
- ethics
- insight
- emotion
- tact
- inhibition
- sequencing thoughts
- evaluates consequences of actions
- solves intellectual problems
- morality
- motor function

Deficits ACA/MCA
- memory problems
- abstract thinking problems
- judgement problems
- ethical behaviour problems
- emotional problems
- insight problems
- tact problems
- inhibition problems

Broca's area
- expression of speech
- word formation
- articulation
- pronunciation
- voice and speech production

- movement problems, trunk, limbs, eyes
- non-fluent aphasia
- oral apraxia

Table 1.3 contd.

Parietal lobe

Functions
- interpretation of sensory input
- contralateral sensation
  two-point discrimination
  pressure
  weight
  texture
  body interpretation
  orientation
  pain
  proprioception
- recognizes nature of complex
  objects by touch and form

Deficits
- sensory deficits
- unilateral neglect

Temporal lobe

Functions
- auditory area
- Wernicke's area:
  receive and discriminate sounds
  interpretation of sounds
- olfactory area
- detailed memories, especially
  those involving more than one
  sensory modality (dominant
  side)

Deficits MCA and PCA
- Wernicke's aphasia
- comprehension
- repetition of speech
- jargon
- reading comprehension

Occipital lobe

Functions
- visual reception
- visual association
- detects spatial organization of
  vision, shapes, colours, contrasts
- secondary complex visual
  interpretatin
- perception of form and meaning
- eye fixation

Deficits
- visual and interpretive disorders
- contralateral field disorders, e.g.
  quandrantopia/hemianopia
- partial visual field loss
- altered perception

Thalamus

Functions
- sensory and motor pathways contact
  thalamus except olfactory pathways

Deficits
- contralateral hemiplegia
- contralateral hemisensory
  deficits
- vertical and lateral gaze
- central post-stroke pain

Table 1.3 contd.

Hypothalamus

Functions

- autonomic nervous system
  blood pressure
  heart rate
  respiratory rate
  body temperature
  water metabolism
  fluid osmolality
  feeding responses
  physical expression of emotions
  sexual behaviour
  hormone synthesis
- regulates salivation, peristalsis,
  sweating and blood sugar

Deficits

- altered temperature regulation
- altered fluid volume status ->
  diabetes insipidus
- altered blood pressure, heart and
  respiratory rate
- altered feeding patterns
- altered blood sugar regulation
- altered gastric motility

Pituitary

Functions

- endocrine system
- release of oxytocin and vasopressin

Deficits

- altered adrenal cortex functioning
- altered body growth
- thyroid disorders
- breast development and lactation
  disorders
- development of primary and
  secondary sex characteristics
- renal problems -> diabetes insipidus

Basal ganglia

Functions

- production of dopamine
- coordination of muscle movements
  and posture

Deficits

- movement and posture disorders
- tremor
- rigidity
- chorea
- athetosis
- dystonia
- hemiballismus

Midbrain

Functions

- synthesizes dopamine
- protects basal ganglia

Deficits

- motor visual problems
- Parkinsonism
- auditory and visual reflexes
  interrupted

Table 1.3 contd.

Pons

Functions
- transmits information from cerebral cortex to brainstem and between two hemispheres
- sensory pathways pass through pons
- regulates respiratory system

Deficits
- sensory and motor problems
- altered mastication and facial sensations
- altered eye movement and eyelid closure
- altered taste, facial expression, salivation, equilibrium and hearing
- respiratory insufficiency

Medulla

Functions
- blood pressure and respiratory regulation
- maintenance of arousal
- initiation of sleep

Deficits
- persistent vegetative state
- contralateral sensory and motor deficits
- altered postural sense, proprioception, vibration
- respiratory insufficiency
- cardiac/vasomotor dysfunction
- swallowing problems
- head and shoulder movement problems
- tongue movement problems
- salivation and pharyngeal function problems

Cerebellum

Functions
- receives proprioceptive input
- maintains equilibrium
- coordinates automatic movement
- regulates muscle tone

Deficits
- ipsilateral decreased muscle tone
- poor coordination and fine dexterity
- gait ataxia
- intention tremor
- diadochokinesia
- dysmetria
- hypotonia
- asthenia

Chapter 2
Early Management

Occupational Therapy – The Stroke Wheel

The stroke wheel is a schematic overview of the management of stroke. In this diagrammatic form, the issues and considerations are expressed in a series of concentric circles. The circles form a ripple effect showing many

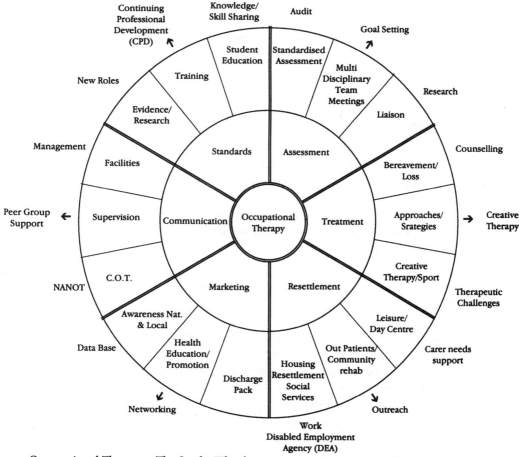

Occupational Therapy – The Stroke Wheel

facets to stroke rehabilitation. The wheel is divided into two halves: the right side focuses on direct patient contact; the left side concentrates on the professional duties. A delicate balance exists as both halves work together, although failure of any of the individual segments (1–6) will impact heavily on the whole service.

Providing a good, effective service is an extremely difficult undertaking, especially with a patient group as diverse as those affected by stroke.

Setting priorities depends very much on the individual therapist; however, it is important to remember the bigger picture. Ideally, consideration should be given to all segments of the wheel. If all these components are working in tandem with each other, the quality of any stroke service will be greatly enhanced.

The wheel represents the breadth of the roles and duties that any therapist working with stroke patients may undertake. Any patient may be represented in any segment of the wheel at any time, and may go through several cycles if he/she changes from one setting to another, for example, acute hospital, rehabilitation centre, community team and social services. The emphasis a particular service puts on each segment of the wheel will vary according to individual need and local practice.

Direct Patient Contact

As may be seen from the stroke wheel, direct contact includes all aspects of patient care. The process may take place in any setting and may involve a number of different agencies.

Assessment includes a variety of standardized and non-standardized measures that inform the occupational therapist about the extent of impairment, disability and handicap. It is important at this stage to understand the patient/carer in relation to his/her cultural and lifestyle needs. Liaison with relatives and/or friends, and other professionals involved in the patient's management, helps to develop a broad picture of the patient and carer and their needs and wants.

Treatment uses the information gained for functional purpose. Treatment techniques are wide and varied depending on the short- and longer-term care aims. Expert help and advice may need to be sought in order to facilitate the best outcome. This may include dealing with loss of roles, identity and adjustment to disability. Whatever type of treatment is offered, it is essential that the exit from this period of intervention is clearly signposted by agreed outcomes, and that a planned move to the next phase of the wheel is understood.

Resettlement This involves returning to the community, and where possible the patient resuming control of his/her own affairs, including work and leisure. The occupational therapist develops a shared responsibility with the patient in helping him/her adjust to residual disability as well as facilitating a return to a meaningful life. Longer-term adjustment may involve social services and voluntary organizations. It is important that carers also have access to ongoing support and advice.

Upon leaving hospital, lifestyle is often changed considerably by the effects of a stroke. Consequently, discharge home with a rail or two and a home carer may not be enough. An individual needs to have choice to be empowered. Resources and facilities, of course, vary from region to region; however, any improvement in the links between hospital and community services can only ease this difficult transition.

Professional Duties

Standards The professional side of the therapist's responsibilities starts with the code of conduct, which confers on the individual the responsibility to provide care of the highest quality possible, within given experience and available local resources.

Government policy has developed in recent years and there is now a demand for evidence to support the clinical effectiveness of our treatments and to keep up to date with new practice. Recommended standards of care are being developed, and as these are implemented there may be training implications for all staff groups. Research is being undertaken into the clinical effectiveness of therapy. The results of the research may lead therapists away from traditional treatment activities into new roles.

Communication This is an increasingly important area, particularly when a therapist finds him/herself working as the only occupational therapist in a multidisciplinary team. In striving for excellence, it is essential to use all of the resources available.

The College of Occupational Therapists has developed tools to help therapists maintain evidence of continued professional development, which will become a requirement under the new Professions Allied to Medicine (PAMS) parliamentary act. Professional supervision is part of the code of conduct, and should be part of everyday practice. The increased use of technology will mean that every occupational therapist has access to the most up-to-date ideas.

Sharing of information is essential to any specialty. This is particularly so in neurology, where innovation and new information affecting practice are constantly appearing. It is therefore important to take the opportunity to enter into dialogue with occupational therapists throughout the country by joining professional groups such as the National Association of Neurological Occupational Therapists (NANOT).

Marketing Promotion of occupational therapy in all its aspects involves informing people about the service they can expect to receive and how to obtain it. In order to provide the best quality service, it is also important that every therapist is aware of local and national policies that could impact on the service. The emphasis away from illness towards healthy lifestyles allows the occupational therapist to develop the health-promotion role.

Frames of Reference/Problem-based Models/Treatment Approaches (Hagedorn, 1992)

Frames of Reference

Definition

A frame of reference is a framework that draws together the underlying theories and hypotheses of an area of study or practice and sets boundaries to, and foundations for, the construction of models and approaches.

Problem-based Models

Definition

A model is a statement of an organized and synthesized body of knowledge that demonstrates relationships between elements within the model and between theory and practice, and coordinates the application of relevant approaches and techniques.

Treatment Approaches

Definition

An approach is a set of ideas and actions that provide the therapist with a particular focus which will lead to the selection of specific assessments, media, treatment techniques, or a style of relationship with the patient.

Frames of Reference (Hagedorn, 1992)

Physiological Frame of Reference

This frame of reference is based on a view of the individual as a biological organism whose behaviour depends on genetically determined factors, combined with the effective action of the nervous and endocrine systems and the ability of the body to maintain homeostasis.

- *The biomechanical approach* is based on kinesiology, which combines neuromuscular physiology, musculoskeletal anatomy and biomechanics.
- *The neurodevelopmental approach* is based on principles of neuromuscular facilitation and sensory integration, and on having a strong developmental base.

Behavioural Frame of Reference

- *The behavioural approach* is primarily a theory of learning, developed from the stimulus response and followed by operant conditioning.

Cognitive Frame of Reference

- *The cognitive approach* is primarily concerned with subjective experiences, i.e. to understand the processes of the mind, such as perception, memory, conceptualization, and to provide theories about how the individual forms relationships between concepts, interprets structures and makes sense of the environment.

Psychodynamic Frame of Reference

This deals with the unconscious motivations for actions, interaction and beliefs, and the symbolic content of images and perceptions.

- *The analytical approach* is derived from psychoanalytical and object relations theories.
- *The interactive approach* is derived from group theory and psychotherapy.

Humanistic Frame of Reference

This is a holistic view of the individual, personal experiences and openness to one's own feelings.

- *The patient-centred approach* encourages the individual to direct his/her own therapy as far as may be possible, to accept personal responsibility and to make decisions.

Problem-based Models (Hagedorn, 1992)

The Rehabilitation Model

Assumes that the patient was previously able, but that function has been lost as a result of illness or injury ('was able, now can't do').

The Developmental Model

Assumes that the patient is not functional because he/she has not yet reached the developmental level which would enable him/her to become so ('is not yet able, can't yet do').

The Educational Model

Views the origin of the problem as being lack of skill, knowledge, appropriate attitude or experience, although the basic ability to become functional is present ('would be able, doesn't know how to').

The Problem-solving Model

Is a description of a process, rather than a set of theories. It is a conscious attempt to avoid the assumptions and blinkered thinking which may be inherent in other models, and to view the patient holistically and objectively before deciding on the nature of the problem and how (or if) to treat it.

Occupational Therapy Models (Hagedorn, 1992)

The Model of Human Occupation (Kielhofner, 1985)

Views a person as an open system interacting with the environment and continually modifying it and being modified by it. The system is arranged as a hierarchy, composed of subsystems; volition (will); habituation (roles, rules); performance (skill).

The Adaptation Through Occupation Model (Reed, 1984; Sanderson and Reed, 1980)

Describes the individual as functioning within the biopsychological, physical and sociocultural environments, continually adapting and providing for his/her needs by means of occupational behaviour in the areas of leisure, self-maintenance and productivity. It defines areas of skill with which the occupational therapist should be concerned, and specifies the assumptions that lie at the heart of the practice of OT.

The Adaptive Skills Model (Mosey, 1981)

Views learnt skills (especially psychosocial ones) and developmental adaptation as the keys to individual function. The structured treatment process relates to the educational/developmental models and is humanistic in outlook, but it also uses elements from behaviourism.

Treatment Approaches (Harrison, 1995)

Neurophysiological

Normal Movement (Bobath)

'It is based on the analysis of normal movement in an individual and the deviation from normal. Direct handling of the body at key points aims to control afferent input and facilitate normal postural reactions. The purpose of this control is to allow patients the experience of normal afferent input and normal movement patterns while inhibiting abnormal afferent input and abnormal movement.' (Bobath 1976, 1990, quoted in Harrison, 1995, p. 6)

'The approach focuses on and aims to control the responses that result from the damaged central postural control mechanism, which is a set of mechanisms that coordinate our postural reactions in all situations. Movements are not isolated to individual joints but take place in patterns. Therapists' handling techniques are interchangeable and require constant adjustment according to the patient's response.'

Brunnstrom

'The approach aims to encourage the return of voluntary movement in patients with hemiplegia through the use of reflex activity and a range of sensory stimulation. The choice of stimulation varies depending on which stage the patient has reached in the motor recovery process.' (Brunnstrom, 1970, quoted in Harrison, 1995, p. 7; see also Sawner and La Vigne, 1992)

'This approach uses primitive reflexes to initiate movement and encourages the use of mass patterns in the early stages of motor recovery. The ultimate aim is for normal function with unwanted activity being controlled at more advanced stages of recovery. Treatment is planned and assessed in stages and movement is encouraged in patterns. The approach does not aim to normalize tone or inhibit the expression of primitive movement.'

Knott and Voss

'This approach aims to promote movement and functional synergies of movement by maximizing peripheral input. Patterns and techniques of proprioceptive neuromuscular facilitation (PNF) are designed to hasten motor learning by providing appropriate sensory stimuli and following activities in a developmental sequence.' (Knott and Voss, 1968, quoted in Harrison, 1995, p. 9; see also Sullivan et al., 1982; Kidd et al., 1992)

'PNF uses peripheral input such as stretch and resisted movements to reinforce existing motor responses. Total patterns of movement are used in treatment and activities are followed in a developmental sequence. The approach does not encourage abnormal movements, unwanted activities are inhibited and problems of abnormal tone are not addressed.'

Rood

'This approach aims to obtain as normal a motor response as possible and, where appropriate, on an automatic level. Sensory stimuli are used to activate or inhibit movement or postural reactions, which are progressed through a developmental sequence.' (Goff, 1969, quoted in Harrison, 1995, p. 10)

'The approach emphasizes the use of activities in a developmental sequence, sensory stimulation and the classification of muscle work. Unwanted activity is inhibited, total patterns of movement are utilized and the aim is for a normal motor response. The approach does not emphasize the use of functional tasks or provide an overall approach to patient management.'

Johnstone

'The main aim of the approach is to control spasticity consistently over time.' (Johnstone, 1980, quoted in Harrison, 1995, p. 11)

'The approach emphasizes the control of spasticity and the facilitation of movement while tone is being controlled. Treatment focuses on the trunk, with total body movements progressing from rolling through to crawling. Family involvement is encouraged. The approach does not utilize abnormal movements.'

Theories of Learning

Peto (Conductive Education)

'This approach aims to teach individuals strategies for dealing with problems of physical disability in order to encourage the child or adult to learn to live with or overcome disability in everyday life. It also aims to provide a totally integrated approach emphasizing continuity and consistency through the use of a conductor.' (Kinsman et al., 1988, quoted in Harrison, 1995, p. 12; see also Kinsman, 1989; Bower 1993)

'The approach emphasizes the use of educational principles and repetition to facilitate independence of individuals in daily activities. Programmes are highly structured and are controlled by the conductor; patients are encouraged to learn actively rather than be treated. Group work, repetition and task analysis are used to reinforce learning. Manual facilitation is not used as in other approaches and patients guide their own movements through bilateral activities. The approach does not emphasize individual treatment, manipulative guidance for correcting movement or the use of enhancing somatosensory stimuli.'

Movement Science (Carr and Shepherd)

'The aim of the framework is to enable the disabled person to learn how to perform or improve performance of actions critical to everyday life. Emphasis is on utilising theories of learning, in particular the use of practice and knowledge of biomechanics for analysing movements and performance of tasks, to encourage people to learn and self-monitor.' (Carr & Shepherd, 1987, quoted in Harrison, 1995, p. 13)

'The approach emphasizes the practice of functional tasks and the importance of relearning real-life activities that have meaning for patients. Careful biomechanical analysis of movements and tasks is highlighted as key to planning treatment and following context-specific training. The programme does not utilize manual guidance techniques for manipulating movement or providing normal afferent input, thus some unwanted activity may emerge.'

Choice of Treatment Approaches

There is a need for consistency of approach within the treatment team and an awareness that some approaches can conflict. The majority of therapists within the UK base their treatment on the Normal Movement approach, although there is little published evidence on the effectiveness of this approach. Ernst (1990) reviewed the evidence for the use of the neurodevelopmental approach and found that most of the published studies showed that the type of approach used did not influence recovery (Logigian et al., 1983; Dickstein et al., 1986; Lord and Hall, 1986; Basmajian et al., 1987). All these studies compared the neurodevelopmental approach with at least one other approach but all lacked specific information about the actual treatment involved. The studies did not use independent assessors, treatment started late and was of short duration and most had only small sample sizes.

Recently, the Movement Science approach has been adopted by some therapists and others favour the Johnstone approach.

The Normal Movement Approach

Normal movement is a problem solving approach to the assessment and treatment of individuals with disturbances of tone, movement and function, due to a lesion of the central nervous system. (International Bobath Tutors Association, 1996)

Normal movement consists of smooth, efficient and coordinated movement in order to achieve a motor goal. It is the constant interaction between key points to move from one postural set to another. The basis of normal movement comes from the central postural control mechanism (CPCM) which is regulated by the central nervous system.

The CPCM consists of:

- *normal postural tone*: a continuous partial state of muscle contraction which is high enough to resist gravity and low enough to allow selective movement to take place;
- *reciprocal innervation*: this allows the graded action between the agonist and antagonist (e.g. biceps and triceps), giving smooth coordinated movements;
- *patterns of movement*: sequences of selective movement in an appropriate alignment for the achievement of a goal;

- *balance reactions*:
    - *equilibrium reactions*: automatic adaptations of postural tone in response to gravity and displacement;
    - *righting reactions*: sequences of selective movements in patterns in response to displacement. Functionally they allow the loss and regaining of midline through trunk righting, head righting, stepping reactions and protective extension of the upper limbs.

Patients are facilitated to experience normal movement on the basis that the patient with central nervous system damage does not learn movement, but the sensation of movement. This results in sensations of normal tone and movement going up to the brain and spinal column, resulting in adaptation of brain matter. This adaptation is called *neuroplasticity*.

Useful Terms

- *Base of support*: This refers to the supporting surface, the body part in contact with it and the relationship between the two. In order to accept the base of support, a person needs movement to relate to it and use it as a reference point.
- *Centre of gravity*: A constant downwards force with which man must develop the ability to interact, in order to move selectively. It is constant and the effect is felt if displaced.
- *Postural set*: An alignment of key points in relation to an accepted base of support.
- *Key points*: Areas of the body where postural tone can most easily be changed. Each key point provides a large source of proprioceptive input to the central nervous system.
  These are points from which it is easier to:
  (a) facilitate and control movements;
  (b) alter postural tone.
- *Associated reactions*: Pathological increases in tone, in response to a stimulus, which are beyond the person's level of inhibitory control. They reflect a loss of reciprocal innervation.

Treatment

Occupational therapists have a key role in re-educating normal movement in all daily living activities, in the rehabilitation of stroke patients.

It is important to be able to analyse the deviation from normal in each individual, including determining the triggers which may produce associated reactions, in order to manage them and prevent their establishment. This can be elicited through retraining with a combination of automatic and volitional routes (often automatic routes are more successful in patients with cognitive problems, by tapping into previously stored movement patterns).

Normal movement is achieved through appropriate handling and facilitation of normal movement patterns in all activities of daily living, in order to ensure the correct interplay between key points as the person moves from one set to another. Normal movement also considers the person's sensory, cognitive and perceptual functioning, and uses goal-orientated and automatic activity.

Treatment Principles

- *Based on analysis of normal movement and the deviation from normal in activities of daily living.*
- *Observation and analysis of movement patterns.*
- *Facilitation of automatic reactions*, i.e. balance: righting/equilibrium reactions, which form a basis of normal movement.
- *Appropriate handling* by therapist to facilitate the experience of normal movement and sensory feedback.
- *Use of appropriate feedback*: Verbal input to provide feedback and to facilitate volitional activity and non-verbal feedback to gain automatic activity and sensory/motor feedback.
- *Inhibition of abnormal movement* and abnormal tone (including associated reactions) to reduce compensation.
- *Bimanual activity* (interplay of both sides of the body) and appropriate positioning and awareness of parts of the body.
- *Grading activity and careful management of effort* to reduce the development of associated reactions and spasticity.
- *Repetition and practice* of motor skills to promote skill acquisition and goal achievement, and to promote carryover into activities of daily living.

How Can Occupational Therapists Use the Principles of Normal Movement in Improving Functional Ability?

Preparation

- Think about how you do daily activities.
- Prior to session take time to plan and analyse treatment strategy.

Good knowledge/awareness of normal movement is necessary to analyse deviation from the normal.

Activity Analysis

When carrying out in-depth activity analysis of normal movement components of a functional task, consider:

- relationship of key points in all movements from one postural set to another;

- alignment;
- automatic, preparation etc.;
- effects of displacement on balance;
- ability to transfer weight;
- selective movement;
- patterns of selective movement required for the task;
- sensation and proprioception;
- cognitive/perceptual demands of the task;
- retained skills, previously stored automatic movement;
- righting reactions needed.

Normalize tone before you start and monitor as you progress

Some preparation may be needed prior to the activities of daily living.

Think about positioning

Consider:

- self in relation to patient — 'Do not over handle';
- teaching patients correct positioning, increasing their autonomy;
- relation to postural sets and skills acquisition.

Assessment of patients in relation to their tone and stamina

This should be done before, during and after each treatment session. Work within their tolerance limits with regard to speed and activity, stamina, concentration and level of activity.

Grading

This relates to:

- length of sessions;
- activity tolerance;
- muscle strength and selective control.

Goal-orientated approach

Negotiate patients' goals with them. Do not be prescriptive.

Be creative in treatment/meaningful activities

Think how normal movement principles can be used in all aspects of patient's life, e.g. ironing, getting on/off bus, running the bath, etc.

Clear visual/verbal instructions as required and proprioceptive feedback

Explain (a) why doing this activity with patient and (b) benefits; give a clear framework; increase their motivation and participation.

Use of equipment

Use equipment to complement normal movement patterns/compensation. 'Normal activity' does not utilize aids to independence other than as a last resort. Aids may be used to minimize effort and disability.

Carryover and skill acquisition

Practice and repetition increase skills learning. Consider:

- carryover between sessions;
- teaching carer to monitor;
- ward staff involvement;
- visual/written instruction;
- teaching skills in a variety of environments;
- if possible teach skills in most appropriate environment to increase carry-over.

Encourage patients to take responsibility

Patients should be encouraged to take responsibility for monitoring abnormal tone — this can be seen as mini goal-setting.

The Movement Science Approach

An overview of the Movement Science Approach based on the observations of Carr and Shepherd (1987), Fellows of the Australian College of Physiotherapy, is highlighted.

This approach presents a shift away from facilitation of movement and exercise therapy, to involving specific training of muscle activity. It is about the functional movement of the affected limbs and the prevention of compensatory activity by *either* the *affected* or *intact* side. Carr and Shepherd also focus on the underactivation of muscle rather than the overactivity affecting movement. The term 'spasticity' is not used in the same context as Bobath, but as loss of muscle elasticity caused by overactivation of muscle groups.

Carr and Shepherd believe all patients are individuals, with basic motor needs common to all. The retraining of motor control is based on an understanding of the 'kinematics' and 'kinetics' of normal movement and the analysis of motor dysfunction, and involves theories of learning and motivation. The emphasis of the approach is based on the training of specific movement components and the conscious elimination of all unnecessary muscle activity.

Carr and Shepherd have identified the essential components required to perform a task and the possible compensations that occur. These essential components, when linked together correctly, allow smooth controlled movement. Four 'tasks' that have relevance to Occupational Therapy are:

1. sit to stand;
2. postural adjustments (balance);
3. reaching and manipulation;
4. walking.

Everyday activities such as drinking from a cup have 'movement components'. The essential components of manipulation are:

- radial deviation combined with wrist extension;
- wrist extension and flexion while holding an object;
- palmar abduction and opposition at the carpo-metacarpal joint of the thumb;
- flexion and opposition of individual fingers towards the thumb;
- flexion and extension of the MCP joints of the fingers with IPs in some flexion;
- supination and pronation of the forearm while holding an object.

Should one or more of the above components be absent or impaired, it will affect the ability to pick up a cup to drink or to use a knife/fork efficiently. The approach lends itself to any task, for example, eating, dressing, kitchen tasks, leisure, transfers, and is based on activity analysis principles.

This approach also has implications for the early provision of splints. Some research conducted suggests that immobilization of muscles in a short-ened position (e.g. wrist flexion, elbow flexion, MCP and IP flexion), a common position of an inactive limb, reduces muscle-fibre length and a loss of serial sarcomeres. It has been found that periods of stretch, as short as 30 minutes, prevent muscle atrophy associated with muscle stiffness. Passive stretching can prevent connective tissue remodelling and muscle stiffness. This and joint stiffness are common causes of pain and reduced range of movement.

The Movement Science Approach links cognitive and motor theory into a holistic analysis of an individual's overall performance, encouraging the patient to be an active participant. The emphasis is on consistency of practice, motivation and repetition of everyday tasks, 'aiming to assist patients to gain their maximum functional potential' (Carr and Shepherd, 1987). This links well with the occupational therapist's skill in activity analysis and with our core skills.

Further Reading

Carr A, Shepherd R. A Motor Relearning Programme for Stroke. London: Heinemann Physiotherapy, 1987. [ISBN 0 433 05152 3]

Ada L, Canning C. Key Issues in Neurological Physiotherapy. London: Heinemann Medical, 1990. [ISBN 07 506 000 98]

Initial Assessment: General Checklist

Aims

- To identify with patient the effects of his/her injury/illness.
- To identify problems and areas of function affected.
- To assess likely effectiveness of intervention.

What Do We Assess?

- Any differences from 'normal'.
- Expected effects of condition impacting on functional performance and ADL.
- Social background/support network.
- Psychological adjustment/impairment.
- Motivation/expectations of therapy.
- Positive aspects.
- Cognitive/perceptual/behavioural impairment.
- Communication/relationships.

Tools of assessment

- Observation.
- Intervention.
- Physical assessment.
- Standardized tests.

What Makes a Good Assessment?

Interview skills

- Establish rapport.
- Therapist approach and beliefs.
- Preparation:
  - collect information;
  - set interview goals;
  - set interview boundaries and time limit.

Format

- Introduction
  - establish rapport;
  - explain your role.
- Use open questions initially, for example:
  - What are your main problems?
  - How do they affect you?
  - Who? What? Where? When?
- Use closed questions to direct interview and gain specific information.
- Give feedback.
- Summarize main points.
- Close interview and give information on next step of process.

What Do We Assess?

The object of assessment is how the physical, social and psychological effects of the stroke impact upon the person's functional ability and their family.

- *Social history*: family relationships, roles, lifestyle, work, carers, support network.
- *Past medical history*: other medical conditions e.g. heart condition, orthopaedic problems.
- *Environmental considerations*: accommodation, layout and adaptations.
- *Functional ability*: personal ADL, domestic ADL, mobility, transfers, etc.
- *Physical sensory difficulties*: tonal problems, hemiplegia, pain, sensory problems.
- *Cognitive problems*: short-term memory problems, concentration, attention, planning, initiation.
- *Perceptual difficulties*: body image, dyspraxia, agnosia.
- *Communication*: dysarthria, expressive/receptive dysphasia.
- *Psychological*: feelings about themselves and others, mood, lability, adjustment to disability.
- *Motivation/Attitude*: realistic.

Physical Assessment Guidelines

The assessment and analysis of patients' problems set the scene for treatment. There is no formal assessment procedure; the idea is to build up a picture of the patient as a whole, and how he/she moves. This is achieved through observation and handling.

Assessments provide us with information for setting goals, both long and short term, in conjunction with other team members. Assessments will, however, provide us with information from which we can get a baseline for treatment. In the assessment the therapist needs to observe the patient move/attempt movement and to feel the patient move.

During the assessment ask yourself:

1. *How does the patient move?*
- Does the patient move but with effort?
- Is the movement disjointed or fluent?
- Are there associated reactions present?
- Can the patient actually move at all?
- How are the movements different from normal?
- Remember to take the ageing process, regarding premorbid posture, into account.

2. *Why does the patient move in this way?*
- Is it tone? High, low, fluctuating, adaptable?
- Are there associated reactions? Upper limb and lower limb.
- Is it due to problems with the underlying balance mechanism?
- Are there sensory problems leading to poor feedback (loss of proprioception, loss of touch)?
- Is there loss of active, selective movement?
- Are there perceptual problems (dyspraxia, neglect/inattention)?

Physical Neurological Assessment

Remember that the patient needs to be suitably undressed for your assessment. You can use their undressing as part of the assessment. Note especially that handling and observation are key to an accurate assessment ('feel' is the term we use for physically assessing changes in tone with your hands and assessing the patient's active and passive range of movement):

If the patient arrives in a wheelchair then have a look at them in this position first:
- What does the head do?
- Feel their trunk. Can they change or maintain position?
- Feel their arms. Is their unaffected arm free to move; is there pain?
- How is their arm positioned? Heavy, light, subluxation, active movement?
- Feel the hips. Restricted, stiff, or floppy?
- Feel the legs. Heavy or light?
- Feel the feet. Mobile, stiff, or sensitive?

Transfers:
- How do they get from the chair to the bed? Independently? Presence of associated reactions? With help?
- How do they get from sitting to lying?

- How do they get from sitting to standing?

Sitting on plinth:
- Sitting unsupported. Can they achieve this? Posture?
- Weight-bearing. Is it symmetrical?
- Overall posture. Can they adapt their posture when handled?
- Posture of legs. Falling in? Pulled out?
- Position of pelvis. Anterior or posterior tilt?

Trunk:
- Can they take their weight laterally?
- Are righting reactions evident?
- Are there areas of high or low tone?
- What is the position of their scapulae?

Upper limb:
- Feel the arms. Heavy, light, uncoordinated?
- Any tight structures, e.g. pectorals, latissimus dorsi, subluxed?
- Pain?
- View from anterior and posterior aspect. What is scapula doing? Rotated, winging, retracted, elevated?
- Is there selective activity in the limb? Is it functional? Can they follow? Can they place?
- Feel the hand. Is it functional? Is it tight? Does it move? Are there soft tissue changes?

Lying:
- Has their tone changed?
- Has their posture changed? Look at position of:
  - head
  - shoulder
  - trunk
  - pelvis

Lower limbs — gait or wheelchair independence:
- Have a good look at patient walking.
- Look at each key point in turn:

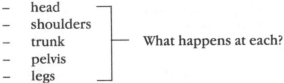

  - head
  - shoulders
  - trunk ⎯ What happens at each?
  - pelvis
  - legs
- Is the head free to move or being held to one side or fixed in the middle?
- Are the shoulders free to move?
- Is there active arm swing or are associated reactions present?

- Is there interaction between both sides of the trunk, righting reactions present?
- What is the orientation of the pelvis?
- What happens to the leg in the stance phase, and in the swing phase?
- What are the feet doing?
- Does the patient use an aid? Does the patient need this aid?

Wheelchair:
- Can the patient self-propel?
- Does he/she remember brakes?
- Is there evidence of associated reactions?
- Is he/she aware of his/her position in preparation when transferring?

Sensation

Sensory loss inhibits motor function even with good motor return, and the inclination to move is based on sensory input and feedback.

Assessment

It is necessary to make sure patient's vision is occluded and test both impaired and normal side. Stimuli are applied in an unpredictable pattern.

Superficial

- *Light touch*: hand and forearm are touched lightly with cotton wool at random locations. After each stimulus the person is asked to respond by saying yes or no.
- *Deep sensation*: as above but press harder.
- *Pain*: affected hand and forearm are touched lightly at random locations using sharp or dull stimuli, e.g. using a pin. Patient should be asked to say 'sharp' or 'dull' in response to each stimulus.
- *Temperature*: use test tubes filled with cold and hot water and touch side of tubes on skin surfaces in random order and random locations.

Stereognosis

This is the ability to recognize objects by touch. It appears to be a perceptual skill that makes it possible to identify common objects and geometric shapes through tactile perception without the aid of vision. Intact stereognosis makes it possible to identify the surface of an object through touch, shape, size and consistency.

To test, occlude patient's vision and ask him/her to feel objects placed in the hand, e.g. pencil, pen, glasses, key, coin.

Proprioception

This is the unconscious awareness of the information from muscles, tendons, ligaments and joints. Conscious awareness occurs when attention is focused.

To test, hold the limb laterally to avoid tactile or pressure input and place the joints of one extremity into easily describable positions. The patient should imitate each position with the opposite limb or describe the position.

The Nottingham Sensory assessment (Lincoln et al., 1991) may be useful. Also a new assessment of sensory awareness has recently been developed called the Rivermead Assessment of Somatosensory Performance (Winward et al., 2000).

Treatment

It is necessary to make the patient aware of the sensory loss and encourage some use of the limb in functional tasks, to improve sensory feedback. If there is limited movement, encourage placing in tasks and weight transference.

In terms of remedial activities, repetition and variation of sensory stimuli are necessary if the patient is to re-learn sensation. He/she can initially do activities with vision present and then move to vision occluded. Systematic retraining can lead to significant gains several years after stroke.

Compensatory techniques include testing water with the other hand, using adaptive devices for safety and training the patient to check the position of his/her limbs.

Carey (1995) reviewed the evidence on the nature and implications of sensory loss in terms of function. Carey found that 50% of stroke patients experience sensory impairment, in particular tactile and proprioceptive discrimination. This had a negative effect on 'exploration of environment, safety, movement and rehabilitation outcomes'. Carey explained that research had shown that somatosensory retraining was effective when neurophysiological and learning concepts were used. Clinically and statistically significant improvements had been found in the discrimination of trained and generalized stimuli.

Functional Assessment

When meeting the patient for the first time it is useful to have considered what you need to know and how you are going to assess it.

Functional assessment of the patient's abilities should include a full screen of previous lifestyle and current abilities. If the patient is able to participate, a discussion about his/her expectations will help guide the choice of intervention.

A full physical examination can be carried out during a functional activity such as washing, dressing or kitchen work.

The therapist should summarize the physical assessment, including how these deficits will affect functional tasks; for example, poor balance mechanisms will affect the patient's ability to dress.

The therapist should then discuss these results with the patient and explain how occupational therapy can improve function.

The use of standardized assessments such as the Canadian Occupational Performance Measure (COPM) (Law et al., 1991) and the Assessment of Motor and Process Skills (AMPS) (Fisher, 1999), are helpful in both planning intervention and measuring its effectiveness.

Goal Setting

Goal Planning

This is a systematic process of identifying needs and planning specific goals and working towards these goals whilst simultaneously evaluating progress and practice.

Benefits for the patient

The major benefit to the patient and carer is that the patient is involved in planning his/her rehabilitation at the beginning and routinely throughout its duration. This increases active participation of the patient and the likelihood of meeting his/her needs. Goal planning also gives patients specific targets and direction, allowing them to break down a general aim or desire into achievable components.

Benefits to the rehab team

These include those mentioned above as benefits to the patient, mainly active participation and direction and motivation. The goal-planning process brings the team together on a regular basis to facilitate a coordinated approach to service provision. The process of planning both long-term and short-term goals allows the team to identify clearly the predicted outcome of their intervention and simultaneously evaluate the effectiveness of their intervention or practice. By evaluating and recording the achievement of the goals the team can provide information relating to clinical outcome.

The brain is goal/function orientated, not movement orientated. Goals need to be patient centred and meaningful, and therefore based on activities of daily living. Repetition and practice are key to skill acquisition. To achieve carryover tasks need to be practised in a variety of environments to achieve a permanent change in behaviour.

Writing Down Goals

When writing down goals, these should reflect the same qualities as any other objective.

They should be SMART:
- Specific;
- Measurable;
- Achievable;
- Realistic;
- Timely.

To measure whether there is a change in behaviour, the goal must be written down as something that can be seen, heard, or counted. In attempting to write a SMART goal, consider: Who...will be doing what — Under what conditions — To what degree of success — Within what period of time? Goals should then be evaluated and reviewed.

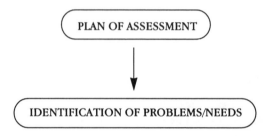

E.G. ARTHUR REQUIRES ASSISTANCE FROM TWO PEOPLE TO WALK OUTDOORS

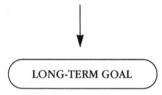

E.G. ARTHUR WILL BE ABLE TO WALK TO AND FROM THE NEWSAGENT X 3/7 TO BUY A NEWSPAPER (LTGs MAY COVER SEVERAL PROBLEMS, E.G. COMMUNICATION, ORIENTATION, MOBILITY)

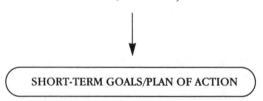

E.G. ARTHUR WILL BE ABLE TO WALK FROM HIS FRONT DOOR TO HIS GARDEN GATE AND BACK WITH ASSISTANCE FROM HIS MOTHER BY 1 FEBRUARY 1997. E.G. TEACHING SESSIONS WITH ARTHUR'S MOTHER RE: HOW TO SUPPORT HIM WHEN WALKING OUTSIDE

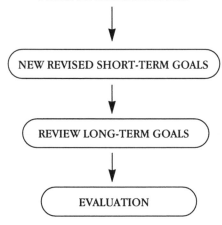

E.G. ARTHUR WILL BE ABLE TO WALK SUPERVISED FROM HIS FRONT DOOR TO THE POSTBOX INDEPENDENTLY

The Use of Standardized Assessments in Clinical Practice

Standardized Assessment

A standardized assessment is one that has an established procedure for its administration, norm scores collected from a representative population, a developed scoring procedure and evidence of the validity and reliability of the assessment.

Considerations when Choosing an Assessment

Many aspects need to be considered when deciding which standardized assessment to use. These include:

- how easily the assessment is obtained;
- whether it is validated for OTs to administer;
- which patients the test has been designed for;
- what evidence is available on its validity;
- what evidence is available on its reliability;
- whether there are norms for comparison;
- the cost of the test;
- how easy is it to administer the test;
- how easy is it to score and interpret the test results;

- whether there is any training needed;
- how easy it is to transport the test;
- what space is needed to administer the test;
- how much time is needed to administer the test;
- what the advantages of the test are;
- what the disadvantages of the test are.

Administering the Test

Again, there are many aspects to consider when administering a standardized assessment, apart from just completing the assessment. These include:

- ensuring that you are familiar with the assessment;
- understanding what you are assessing and why;
- checking whether patient needs glasses, hearing aid, toilet etc.;
- checking that patient understands why you are doing the assessment;
- having the room prepared: quiet, without interruptions, suitable furniture etc.;
- having the assessment materials ready and out of direct sight of patient;
- having a clipboard available to record scores on, out of sight of patient;
- recording also any details of behaviour and types of errors made during the assessment;
- not using individual sections of a test alone, unless the instructions say this is valid;
- ensuring that you adhere to the words and demonstration given in the manual/instructions;
- not giving the patient any additional information about the test until it is completed;
- not telling the patient how he/she is performing during the test; wait until it is completed;
- being aware of your body language; this could affect the results obtained;
- considering dysphasic patients — can they follow the instructions?;
- considering the effects of other impairments on the patient's performance on this particular assessment;
- after completion of the test, explaining the results and impairments to the patient, with relevance to his/her situation in functional terms and what treatment you can offer for these impairments.

Other Impairments

Other impairments could affect the patient's ability to complete the assessment being carried out. These could include:

- whether he/she is using his/her non-dominant hand;
- language ability;

- comprehension ability;
- concentration and attention levels;
- initiation ability;
- presence of dyspraxia;
- reasoning ability;
- memory loss;
- presence of depression;
- presence of anxiety;
- hemianopia or diplopia;
- general eyesight;
- overall effect of inattention.

Interpreting Results

When interpreting the results of an assessment, consider whether there is any evidence of these impairments causing an impact on the patient's functional ability. Also, consider whether it is preferable in that patient's situation to do the assessment before or after a functional assessment and whether any difficulties arise. Do not use a standardized assessment instead of a functional assessment of the patient's abilities – both are needed.

Standardized ADL Assessments

There are many standardized activities of daily living (ADL) assessments available for use with stroke patients and yet it is still difficult to find one that is suitable for some needs.

The following are considerations concerning some of the ADL measures already developed and available:

- *Barthel ADL Index* (Mahoney and Barthel, 1965; Collin et al., 1988). Although well recognized and well used, this assessment does not include bed mobility, kitchen or household activities. Each item is graded but there are varying numbers of grades for each item and different maximum scores, i.e. 0–1, 0–2, 0–3. The total score only is frequently used by the medical profession.
- *Rivermead ADL assessment* (Whiting and Lincoln, 1980; Lincoln and Edmans, 1990). This is a ranked assessment measuring self-care and household activities. The scoring for each item is dependent, verbal assistance only or independent and therefore does not show changes in the degree of dependence or how much help is required.
- *Nottingham 10-point ADL scale* (Ebrahim et al., 1985). This is a 10-point ranked assessment, including mainly self-care activities. Each item is scored as dependent or independent and again therefore does not show changes in the degree of dependence or how much help is required.

- *Northwick Park ADL index* (Benjamin, 1976). This index also measures mainly self-care activities. Each item is scored as dependent, partially dependent or independent and as before does not therefore show changes in the degree of dependence or how much help is required.
- *Australian ADL index* (Spencer et al., 1986). This is a modification of the Northwick Park ADL index with similar scoring, except each item is graded 1–3 instead of dependent, partially dependent or independent. As before, this scoring shows insufficient changes to monitor progress in clinical practice.
- *Sheikh et al. modified ADL index* (Sheikh et al., 1979). This index is also a modification of the Northwick Park ADL index with scoring and limitations as for the Australian ADL index.
- *Edinburgh Stroke study* (Smith, 1979). This assessment has good grades of scores, ranging from 1 to 7, but does not include activities in much detail.
- *Functional Independence Measure (FIM)* (Granger et al., 1986). This measure includes mainly self-care activities and has limited evidence of reliability.
- *Frenchay activities index* (Holbrook and Skilbeck, 1983; Wade et al., 1985). This index assesses premorbid ability and is designed for use with outpatients. It is unsuitable for inpatients.
- *Nottingham extended ADL scale* (Nouri and Lincoln, 1987). This ADL scale again was designed for use with outpatients and includes many activities unsuitable for patients to carry out in hospital.
- *Katz ADL Index* (Katz et al., 1963). This index includes six items only and is graded according to how many items the patient is independent in. As with previous indices it does not therefore show changes in the degree of dependence or how much help is required.
- *Kenny self-care assessment scale* (Schoening et al., 1965). This scale is graded from 0 to 4 and is aimed at nursing-care requirements but does not include activities for life outside hospital.
- *Pulses profile* (Granger et al., 1979). This profile is intended to be used with the Barthel ADL index and does not include much detail on individual items.
- *Edmans ADL index* (Edmans and Webster, 1997). This is a new index, published in October 1997. Scoring on each item is 0–3 and it was designed to include all activities necessary to enable a person to live independently at home, and to be able to monitor progress in patients' abilities over time.

Eakin (1989a) gave an excellent review of ADL assessments and described three types of ADL assessment:

1. *Check list* – which describes but does not measure performance and often has no scoring.
2. *Summed index* – where each item is scored to give a total. However, if each item is scored equally, there is the assumption that each has the same disability value, i.e. is the ability to climb stairs or have a bath of equal disability? On a 20-point scale, is a change from five to ten of the same importance as a change from 15 to 20? Such assessments therefore need to be interpreted carefully.
3. *Hierarchical scale* – where tests are passed in a particular order for all patients.

In another paper, Eakin (1989b) also discussed the requirements of an ADL assessment. She suggested the following:

> The assessment should be representative, i.e. the activities should reflect the activities of a patient's normal life. The activities included should be relevant and sensible, providing the information required only, i.e. no more and no less. The activities should also measure what they are intended to measure, to achieve the purpose required.

The assessment should be reliable, i.e. the result of the assessment should be due to a change in the patient's performance and not due to any other factors, for instance, a difference between assessors. It should also be sensitive enough to detect the differences expected or required.

The results should be meaningful to others, i.e. it should be possible to understand and to compare the results of the assessment. The results should be able to be communicated to others and should be simple enough to use.

Positioning for the Early Stroke Patient

People are dynamic, moving individuals and when positioning it is important to consider the functional activities an individual wishes to achieve, in any given posture. In the early stages of recovery, when movements are restricted by the effects of their stroke, individuals are unlikely to be able without assistance to make the postural adjustments required to maintain a symmetrical posture. There are basic principles that can be followed to allow the individual to perform desired activities while assisting in the recovery process. These principles will help recovery by maintaining a passive range of movement, allowing the individual to use the control he/she has and providing normal sensory and proprioceptive input.

The Bed

The bed, in the initial stages following stroke, is the position where the individual is most incapacitated. An inability to roll, or change position without help or extreme effort, leaves him/her with little control over his/her environment. Those with sensory loss on the hemiplegic side may fear turning, or lying on the affected side, while lying on the unaffected side restricts the use of the sound upper limb. Often the individual is nursed on his/her back, which can restrict visual fields and may leave the individual unable to use his/her upper limb.

There are advantages to the individual spending time in bed in that it is the position of fullest support. Those with high tone may benefit from returning to bed for periods during the day to help manage tone. Similarly, those with low tone may be fatigued by the effort required to maintain their posture against gravity, and may need rest periods to be built into their day. Correct positioning for sleeping and the early development of functional bed mobility are advised.

How to position in bed

Support should be offered where required to enable the individual to maintain his/her position; in side-lying this may include support along the back to prevent rolling onto the back, and to offer proprioceptive indicators to the hemiplegic side. When the individual is lying on the affected side the affected arm may be placed outstretched, with the shoulder protracted. The

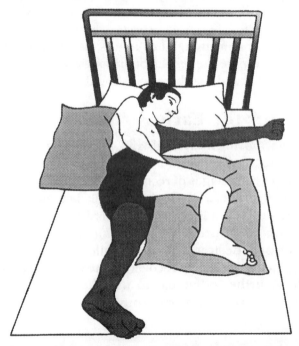

Figure 2.1 Positioning in bed, lying on the affected side (left hemiplegic patient). Do ensure: (i) affected shoulder is brought through, (ii) affected leg is extended at hip and slightly fixed at knee. (iii) there are no objects in the hand or against the sole of the foot, (iv) head is in line with the body.

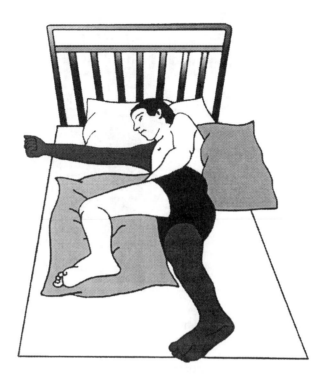

Figure 2.2 Positioning in bed, lying on the affected side (right hemiplegic patient). Do ensure: (i) affected shoulder is brought through, (ii) affected leg is extended at hip and slightly fixed at knee, (iii) there are no objects in the hand or against the sole of the foot.,(iv) head is in line with the body.

lower limb should be slightly flexed with the unaffected side bent over the leg; if necessary a pillow should be placed under the knee to reduce any adductor tone developing (see Figures 2.1 and 2.2).

When lying on the unaffected side the position is reversed; however, the individual who is unable to roll independently will be more incapacitated in this position, so the call bell must be within reach (see Figures 2.3 and 2.4). Side-lying on the unaffected side is a position of choice for at least some of the time for those who have an overactive sound side. In this position they receive proprioceptive feedback about the midline, elongation of the trunk on the sound side is facilitated and weight bearing through the overactive side is promoted.

When positioning an individual on his/her back, it may be necessary to use pillows to prevent the affected shoulder and hip falling into retraction. Lying on the back is also a good position to allow the pectoral muscles to be stretched with the arm supported in abduction (see Figures 2.5 and 2.6). Similar support will be necessary for patients sitting up in bed (see Figures 2.7 and 2.8).

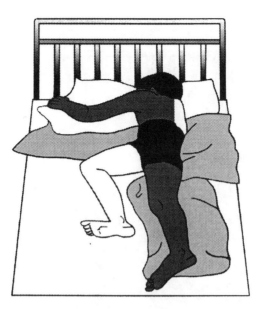

Figure 2.3 Positioning in bed, lying on the unaffected side (left hemiplegic patient). Do ensure: (i) patient's head is in line with the body, (ii) patient is in full side lying not quarter turn, (iii) body is not twisted. (iv) affected shoulder is brought through,(v) arms are kept parallel, unaffected arm **under** pillow, (vi) fingers in a neutral position. Do **not** place any object in the hand or against the sole of the foot.

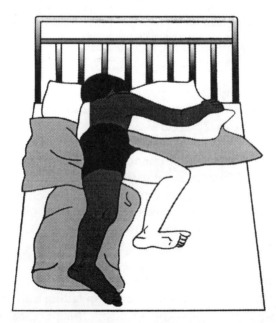

Figure 2.4 Positioning in bed, lying on the unaffected side (right hemiplegic patient). Do ensure: (i) patient's head is in line with the body, (ii) patient is in full side lying not quarter turn, (iii) body is not twisted, (iv) affected shoulder is brought through, (v) arms are kept parallel, unaffected arm **under** pillow, (vi) fingers in a neutral position. Do **not** place any object in the hand or against the sole of the foot.

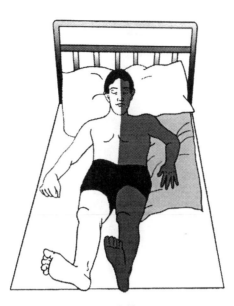

Figure 2.5 Positioning in bed, lying on the back (left hemiplegic patient). Do ensure: (i) head is in the middle, (ii) trunk is elongated on affected side ,(iii) shoulder is kept forward by a pillow, (iv) pillow is under hip to prevent retraction of the pelvis and lateral rotation of leg. Do **not** place any object in the hand or against the sole of the foot.

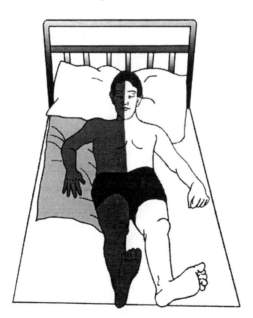

Figure 2.6 Positioning in bed, lying on the back (right hemiplegic patient). Do ensure: (i) head is in the middle, (ii) trunk is elongated on affected side, (iii) shoulder is kept forward by a pillow, (iv) pillow is under hip to prevent retraction of the pelvis and lateral rotation of leg. Do **not** place any object in the hand or against the sole of the foot.

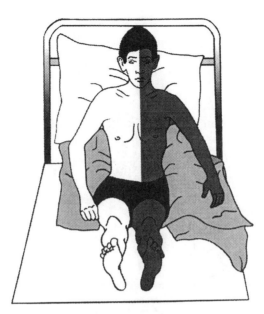

Figure 2.7 Positioning in bed, sitting up in bed (left hemiplegic patient). Do ensure: (i) the patient is upright with **weight evenly distributed on both buttocks**, (ii) shoulder is protracted away from side and forward on a pillow, (iii) legs are straight and not laterally rotated. Do **not** place any object in the hand or against the sole of the foot.

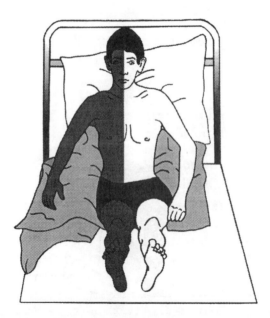

Figure 2.8 Positioning in bed, sitting up in bed (right hemiplegic patient). Do ensure: (i) the patient is upright with **weight evenly distributed on both buttocks**, (ii) shoulder is protracted away from side and forward on a pillow, (iii) legs are straight and not laterally rotated. Do **not** place any object in the hand or against the sole of the foot.

It is important to consider mattresses when positioning the patient. A firm, supportive surface will provide proprioceptive feedback, enable rolling and promote independence when sitting up. However, pressure areas also need to be monitored. Where hospital pressure-care mattresses are used, the patient is likely to require more assistance to turn and sit up.

Encouraging the patient to sit up through side-lying promotes head-righting, weight transference, and a sense of midline.

The Chair

More independence is offered to early stroke patients in supported sitting and they gain a more normal visual perspective of their environment. There is scope for the unaffected arm to be used in a range of functional activities. The trunk muscles begin to be used actively and the lower limbs begin to form a stable base of support.

It is important to note that sitting is not a passive task; the early patient may develop inappropriate muscle activity and 'holding' postures if he/she does not receive sufficient support from the chair or pillows. Those with sensory loss will require pressure areas to be monitored. Where head control is still lacking, support must be provided.

Armchairs generally provide a back support that is slightly reclined; this allows for more relaxation. Where there is little active muscle control, the patient may have a tendency to slide forwards in the chair. This may encourage excess abdominal activity and once established will make active extension difficult.

Provision of a wheelchair allows the patient to be easily transported to different places. A wheelchair provides a more active sitting posture, which encourages greater freedom of upper limb movements. Pressure relief is an important consideration if the person is unable to change position without assistance, but this still needs to provide a stable base.

Points to consider when positioning in a chair

Where possible the individual's hips, knees and ankles should be at 90° flexion with the feet on a firm flat surface. Abduction/adduction of the hip may require wedges to facilitate the correct alignment.

The armrests should allow the arms to be resting on them without the trunk leaning to the side. The arm position may be altered between internal and external rotation at the shoulder, and the forearm between pronation and supination. The arm may also be positioned on a table in front (see Figures 2.9 and 2.10) or to the side of the patient (see Figures 2.11 and 2.12). These variations help to maintain a passive range of movement and prevent shortening of the affected muscle groups. Care should be taken to prevent tightness in the pectoral muscles causing difficulty with dressing in the early stages, and affecting reach in the later stages of recovery. The hand should be maintained in a functional/neutral position, if necessary using resting splints. Web space and rotation of the thumb should be passively maintained, in order to preserve functional viability of the hand.

Perch Sitting

When the patient begins to gain some active sitting balance and transfers are progressing, positioning on a perching stool allows for more active sitting, improving dynamic control of balance, active extension of trunk and weight bearing through lower limbs. The upper limbs are freed to perform a greater range of activities. The extra seat height and position of the pelvis in anterior tilt facilitates easier transfers into the standing position.

Points to consider when using a perching stool

Choose a perching stool with the correct amount of support, e.g. with arms/back rest as appropriate. Ensure the affected hip is not retracted. Both feet should have even weight bearing and should be placed on a firm flat surface.

Sometimes perch sitting is contraindicated as it can exacerbate abnormal patterns of movement/positioning, although it may be the only functional option in the long term.

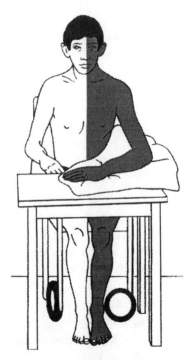

Figure 2.9 Positioning in a chair, affected arm supported in front (left hemiplegic patient). Do ensure: (i) arm is well supported on table/pillows, (ii) the feet are flat on the floor/footplates.

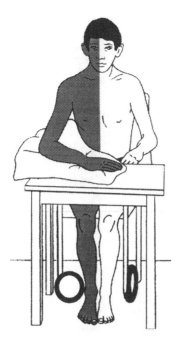

Figure 2.10 Positioning in a chair, affected arm supported in front (right hemiplegic patient). Do ensure: (i) arm is well supported on table/pillows, (ii) the feet are flat on the floor/footplates.

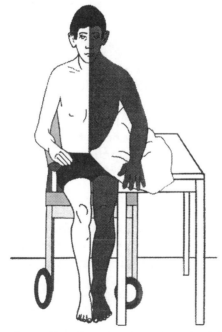

Figure 2.11 Positioning in a chair, affected arm supported at side (left hemiplegic patient). Do ensure: (i) arm is well supported on table/pillows, (ii) the feet are flat on the floor/footplates.

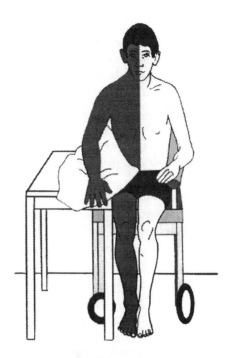

Figure 2.12 Positioning in a chair, affected arm supported at side (right hemiplegic patient). Do ensure: (i) arm is well supported on table/pillows, (ii) the feet are flat on the floor/footplates.

Equipment

The assessment for and provision of equipment to stroke patients is generally viewed as a compensatory method of reducing handicap. Most equipment is issued following a home assessment visit completed prior to weekend leave and/or discharge. However, some equipment can be used to facilitate normal movement and increase independence within the hospital setting. The pros and cons of timing and type of equipment should be carefully considered in conjunction with the patient, family and multidisciplinary team.

Wheelchairs

The provision of a wheelchair for a patient following a stroke can be considered for two main reasons: for correct positioning during early management and for indoor/outdoor mobility during the rehabilitation stage.

The type of wheelchair appropriate for a stroke patient could include attendant-propelled manual wheelchairs and indoor or outdoor powered wheelchairs.

Attendant-propelled manual wheelchairs can be used to achieve better positioning and to improve sitting balance on the ward, which cannot always be possible with armchairs or high-seat chairs. A pressure-care cushion should always be provided with the wheelchair and monitored throughout the day by nursing staff and therapists. Access to attendant-propelled wheelchairs adjusted for specific patients can also enable patients to be taken off the ward by their visitors for often much-needed stimulation. Ideally, a wheelchair should also be available for the patient to use for outdoor and/or indoor mobility on weekend leaves and on discharge. Patients should be discouraged from trying to propel themselves with their feet and self-propelling manual wheelchairs should be avoided altogether. The high-toned patient's muscle tone will increase when using the unaffected arm and leg in this way.

Indoor powered wheelchairs could be considered for patients with severe physical disability and those with chronic heart and lung conditions. A patient's cognition and visual perception should be fully assessed as part of the wheelchair assessment. The use of a powered wheelchair in hospital can help increase motivation and might be considered as a treatment for spatial awareness problems and inattention.

A combined indoor/outdoor and outdoor powered wheelchair would require a full assessment by the hospital-based occupational therapist and wheelchair therapist, carefully taking into consideration the patient's vision, perception and cognition. These wheelchairs can be issued to patients with severe, long-term mobility problems.

When assessing for any type of wheelchair on a long-term basis, the home environment and local area in which the patient will be living should always be taken into account. The access to the patient's home, the type of accommodation, the width of all internal/external doorways, the layout of the furniture and other fixtures/fittings, the door thresholds and the floor coverings should be considered in respect of their suitability for a wheelchair.

ADL Equipment

The provision of equipment by the occupational therapist can assist stroke patients in the following activities of daily living:

- washing/dressing/grooming;
- toileting;
- bathing/showering;
- meal preparation;
- eating.

Washing/dressing/grooming

Long-handled equipment such as a sponge, shoehorn and easi-reach can be useful for patients who have restricted trunk mobility, but should not deter them trying to gain more movement. One-handed equipment such as a suction nail brush and soap holder can be used if a patient does not regain upper limb function but wishes to become more independent in washing. A perching stool can help patients who are unable to stand for prolonged periods whilst carrying out a task or who fatigue easily.

Toileting

Raised toilet seats and frames will encourage a patient to move from sitting to standing in a more normal way than pulling on grab rails fixed to a wall.

Bathing/showering

Many stroke patients with independent sitting balance can manage transfers on and off a bath board, but a bath seat is generally too difficult because of the amount of effort involved. This in turn can increase muscle tone and be too strenuous for people with chronic heart and lung conditions and the frail elderly. Non-slip mats should always be provided or purchased, to be used in conjunction with bath boards/seats. Chairs or seats that fix across the top of the bath for use with a shower, or that lower into the bath, require less effort for the stroke patient and carer and are much safer for those with poor sitting balance. Step-in shower cubicles have limited space for small stools or seats fixed to the wall and are therefore only accessible to the more mobile stroke patient, who can wash him/herself independently whilst standing or sitting on a stool.

Meal preparation

Some kitchen equipment such as large-handled utensils or cutlery issued by occupational therapists could be used by patients with some return of hand function, to encourage further improvement or facilitate more normal movement. These could be used during meal preparation sessions in hospital or at home. Many other pieces of equipment are designed for one-handed use or to make heavy tasks lighter. A spike board, belliclamp, wall-mounted tin opener and buttering board will enable the patient with limited upper limb function to prepare meals. A kettle tipper and cooking basket make dealing with boiling water safer and lighter. A trolley can be used by the more mobile patient to carry hot food.

Fatigue is a major factor to consider when preparing a meal. The layout of the kitchen and its existing equipment or appliances can be looked at during a home assessment visit. Some portable items could be moved closer together in order to conserve the patient's energy. A perching stool could also help reduce fatigue.

Eating

During the acute stage good positioning whilst eating will assist safer feeding and swallowing. Plates that retain heat will keep food warmer for a slow eater. Plateguards and large-handled mugs with lids reduce the risk of spillage. Dycem mats will keep plates in place. Large-handled cutlery could be used with the affected hand to encourage further return of movement. At a later stage, the one-handed patient may require a rocker knife or a fork with a serrated edge for cutting.

Splinting Patients Following Stroke

On reviewing the literature there is a paucity of research and limited consensus of opinion among occupational therapists and physiotherapists on when and how to splint the adult stroke patient. Coppard and Lohman (1996) describe the issue of splinting the neurological upper limb as:

> ...an amorphous quick-sand waiting to engulf the unwary therapist. (p. 195)

In the literature there has been lengthy debate on the theoretical basis for splinting in neurology, that is, whether a biomechanical or neurophysiological approach is used by the therapist. This in turn affects the therapist's reasons for splinting, which can be varied. A splint could be used to reduce flexion contractures, increase range of movement, reduce pain or improve hand function, depending on the type of splint. A wide variety of splint materials and designs have been used: thermoplastics, neoprene, casting and airsplints. Splints may be static or dynamic. There has been considerable discussion in the literature on whether the dorsal or volar surface of the hand should be splinted. The suggested length of time for wearing a splint has also created much debate.

Thermoplastic Splinting

Splinting the neurologically impaired hand following a stroke, as previously mentioned, remains a controversial subject owing to the limited research and contradictory results (Langlois et al., 1989). Thermoplastic splinting is frequently carried out by occupational therapists in their clinical practice. However, before a splint is fabricated, the patient should be assessed on an individual clinical basis by an experienced clinician or under guidance.

Reasons for splinting must be clearly identified, and may include:

* preventing loss of range of movement, associated with altered tone, loss of muscle length and soft tissue changes;
* increasing range of movement;
* relieving oedema;
* improving/maintaining joint alignment;
* maintaining hand hygiene and skin care.

Types of splints most commonly used are the volar splint, dorsal splint, finger spreader, cone (Edwards, 1996) and the palm protector/shield. The literature remains inconclusive and permits no definite conclusions as to which type of splint design is most effective (Langlois et al., 1989). At present there is no clear evidence on the length of time for which a splint should be worn or if it should be worn during the day or night, or during rest periods. A clinician therefore has to make his or her decision regarding type of splint and wearing regime depending on the reason for the splint and the overall goal.

Before splinting, clinicians need to be aware of the Association of Chartered Physiotherapists Interested in Neurology (ACPIN) guidelines on splinting adults with neurological dysfunction. These will assist the clinical decision making, facilitate standardization of clinical management, improve standards of practice and assist the audit process. The guidelines describe the overall assessment and intervention process. Consent should be obtained from the patient/carer, clinical and medical team. Precautions should be identified and if a decision to proceed is made, then a clinical rationale for proceeding should be identified. Documentation should include: area to be splinted, reasons for splinting, type of splint, range of movement, physical appearance, type of materials/padding/strapping and wearing regimes. Written information should be provided for patients/staff and a date of planned review should be identified. Ideally, objective measures should be used to monitor the effectiveness of the splint.

Many questions remain regarding splinting after a stroke, including timing of intervention, type of splint, type of material, wearing regimes and overall effect on spasticity. Clinicians therefore have to make their own decisions using the relevant literature and guidelines available.

Dynamic Lycra Splinting

Second-skin dynamic lycra splints were developed in Australia several years ago. They were designed for two main reasons, for patients following stroke:

1. *For patients who have some return of active movement*: dynamic lycra splints may be used to facilitate return of movement, by their effect on tone, posture and patterns of movement. The patient needs to move and carry out functional activities in the splints for the splints to be of most benefit. These splints encourage the patient to work in biomechanically more efficient postures and using more normalized patterns of movement than static splints allow. Unlike static splints, dynamic lycra splints allow the patient to move throughout a range of postures and patterns of movement during the day.

2. *For those patients with little or no active return of movement*: dynamic lycra splints can be used to reduce pain, oedema and tone and can also be used to improve skin condition. A more relaxed, easily controlled upper

limb facilitates ease of transfers and dressing, and has a positive effect on the patient's gait pattern.

If requested to splint a stroke patient (whether static or dynamic splint), the occupational therapist should consider the reasons very carefully. The patient's diagnosis, level of arousal, pain, sensation, compliance and prognosis should be discussed with the multidisciplinary team. Splinting should not replace any aspect of existing therapy but should form part of a treatment programme. It is recommended that treatment of this nature be discussed with an experienced therapist. The effectiveness of the splint should be evaluated and reviewed on a regular basis. This would require the cooperation of other therapists and nursing staff.

'Splinting in neurology' courses are often organized by occupational therapists and physiotherapists, and give participants the opportunity to fabricate different types of splint and debate the issues surrounding the advantages and problems.

Further Reading

Edwards S. Neurological Physiotherapy: A Problem Solving Approach. Edinburgh: Churchill Livingstone, 1996. [ISBN 0443 04887 8]
Boehme R. Improving Upper Body Control. New York: Psychological Corporation, 1995. [ISBN 0 7616 4137 8]

Further Information

Further information regarding dynamic lycra splinting can be obtained by contacting Jenny Colegate. Tel: (UK) 0131 339 8885.

Chapter 3
Management of
Motor/Sensory Deficits

Therapeutic Aims

The main physical aims of occupational therapy are:

1. to reinforce normal patterns of movement during activity. The patient must be given time to recognize the correct feeling of each movement;
2. to avoid abnormal patterns of movement during activity;
3. to restore as much function as possible to the affected side;
4. to increase independence to enable the patient to return home and lead as normal a life as possible.

Management Principles

Managing Physical Problems

As yet there are no proven rules that identify one treatment approach as better than another. What has been shown to be of most benefit is a coordinated approach between team members treating the patient (National Clinical Guidelines for Stroke, 1999). In Britain the most widely used method of treatment used by neurological therapists is based on the theory developed by Bobath (1976). Introduced widely for physiotherapists in the late 1970s it has become the accepted norm in most hospital-based therapy departments. Subsequent practitioners have further developed the principles of normal movement outlined in this approach.

For the occupational therapist, these principles can be easily incorporated in therapy sessions enhancing the therapy offered to the patient. These principles may be applied in both the hospital and community setting.

In physical management the following principles are applied:

(a) The patient is encouraged to involve the affected side in activities by facilitation.
(b) Associated reactions are avoided through reducing the effort required to move.

(c) The environment is set up to promote the patient's even weight bearing and normal posture and balance.

(d) The therapist, to promote normal movement sequences, facilitates normal activities of daily living, such as self-care and domestic tasks.

(e) Early adaptation of the tasks, to enable independence, should not encourage the patient to adopt abnormal postures.

(f) Tasks may be presented in ways that will challenge the patient's balance mechanisms and encourage novel problem-solving solutions to movement problems.

Self-care Activities

The above management principles should be incorporated in functional activities. Patients should be encouraged to carry out activities in their most normal way. However, in the ward situation patients may have to wash and dress by the side of the bed, which is not the normal experience for most individuals.

Washing

Where possible self-care tasks should be facilitated in the bathroom/washroom or department, where there is more space and access to water and sink etc.

If the patient has sufficient balance, perch sitting allows for greater experience of normal movement and presents the sink at the same height as at home.

Below is a suggested technique for washing:

- The patient should be sitting in a wheelchair, in a chair with arms or on the side of the bed, with a bowl in front of him/her on a low stool (to encourage him/her to lean forwards), or at the washbasin. Alternatively he/she may sit on a perching stool at the washbasin. He/she should aim to maintain sitting balance whilst washing and have wash kit and towel on the affected side to encourage him/her to look to that side.

- Unless the patient has any perceptual deficits, he/she should be able to wash his/her top half except for his/her sound arm and back. To wash under the affected arm he/she should lean forwards, so that the affected arm hangs down straight at the side of his/her affected leg, keeping the affected shoulder protracted. Therapists should consider the effects of a subluxed shoulder and pain during this task.

- To wash his/her lower half, the patient should wash as much as possible whilst sitting, maintaining inhibition of his/her affected arm. When he/she needs to stand, the carer should encourage the correct standing position and balance, so he/she can wash his/her own bottom, retaining his/her dignity. If appropriate, he/she may be able to weight bear through his/her affected hand in standing, while washing his/her bottom. If doing this, great care must be taken not to cause damage to the wrist.

- False teeth may be washed in the washbasin by wedging them in the plughole or using a suction nailbrush stuck to the side of the basin.

Commonly encountered problems in washing include:

(a) difficulty with wringing out a flannel: this may be overcome by using the taps to turn the cloth against or using a small flannel and squeezing it out with one hand;
(b) difficulty putting soap onto a flannel: put soap in a soap dish or on a dry cloth and wipe the flannel over the soap. Alternatively, liquid-soap dispensers can be used;
(c) difficulty cleaning nails: advise use of a suction nailbrush;
(d) getting in/out of bath: use bath board and seat with non-slip mat;
(e) shaving: advise use of electric razor;
(f) cleaning teeth or dentures: use a suction denture brush as a toothbrush or soak dentures in Sterident overnight.

Bathing

A suggested technique for bathing is given below:

- The patient needs to have active sitting balance and be able to lean forwards safely when unattended, before he/she is taught to use the bath board and seat.
- The patient's chair may be positioned alongside the bath. He/she should transfer to sitting on the bath board using his/her usual method of transferring and ensuring that his/her sound side will go in the bath first.
- He/she should move his/her sound leg into the bath, maintaining sitting balance. The carer should then move the affected leg into the bath, ensuring the leg does not hyperextend at the knee. At the same time the carer should keep one arm around the patient's back, maintaining flexion of the patient's trunk and preventing mass extension of the trunk.
- The patient should keep both knees flexed and both feet securely on a non-slip bath mat. The carer should control the affected leg at the knee or ankle and keep one arm around the patient's back for security.
- The patient then puts his/her hand on the side of the bath and gently lowers him/herself down onto the bath seat. The carer must control the affected leg at the knee or ankle to prevent it shooting forwards into extension and must keep one arm around the patient's back, keeping the affected shoulder protracted and ensuring safety. The patient is allowed to push on the side of the bath because the carer is breaking the stroke pattern on the affected side, by maintaining the affected leg in flexion. The patient can straighten his/her legs to bathe but must bathe at this level as it

will be too difficult to get out from the bottom of the bath.

- To get out the reverse is done. The carer can assist in moving the patient back onto the bath board by gently moving the affected knee backwards whilst controlling the knee. The patient should be encouraged to lean forwards whilst moving his/her bottom back and up towards the seat. The patient is likely to be anxious when getting out of the bath initially, therefore it is essential to inhibit the stroke pattern at this time.

Dressing

Early independence in dressing can be encouraged by asking the patient to dress the affected side first. Loose-fitting and stretchy fabrics make the task easier to begin with, but the therapist should remember to check the patient's ability to put on his/her usual day clothes.

Adaptations may be made to garments with Velcro, to provide wider openings, or with a long cord attached to zip fastenings to enable them to be pulled up.

A suggested technique for dressing is given below:

- The patient should be sitting on the side of the bed (preferably), in a wheelchair or in a chair with arms. Sitting on the side of the bed will help to improve his/her sitting balance, trunk control and weight transference and gives him/her greater freedom to move.
- His/her position should be assessed throughout dressing, to ensure maintenance of correct positioning.
- The patient should not be allowed to use excess effort, as this will produce associated reactions and increase tone in the affected side.
- All garments should be placed on the affected side of the patient, to encourage him/her to look towards the affected side to pick them up. Patients suffering from unilateral neglect may need the garments to be positioned in front of them initially and gradually moved to the affected side.
- If the patient can be assisted to dress in a standing position, this may be the most automatic posture for him/her.

To put on bra/vest/jumper/dress/shirt/blouse/cardigan/skirt:

The patient should lay the garment on his/her knees so that the back is uppermost; he/she can then easily see which arm goes into which sleeve. The sleeve hole of the affected arm should be positioned so the sleeve hangs down by the affected leg. The patient should move his/her affected hand into the sleeve hole, lean forwards and slide the affected arm down the sleeve. Next he/she should pull the sleeve up past his/her elbow with the sound hand. He/she should then sit up straight, put his/her sound arm into the other sleeve and pull the jumper etc. over his/her head. Some patients may find it easier, when putting a shirt/blouse on, to lay it out with the collar nearest them, the inside of the shirt/blouse uppermost and sleeves corresponding to the appropriate arm. The patient may need reminding that clothes may get stuck on the affected shoulder and may need pulling down. Bras can be put on this way also, providing they are elasticated and are fastened first.

To remove all upper garments:

The patient should gather each garment up from the back of the neck and pull it over his/her head. The arms should be taken out of the sleeves, keeping the affected arm in the correct position.

To put on pants/trousers/socks/stockings/shoes:

The patient should cross his/her affected leg over his/her sound leg, assisting as required. He/she should lean forwards to put each garment over his/her affected foot, keeping his/her affected arm hanging down by the side of his/her affected leg, i.e. in the correct position. He/she should then uncross his/her legs and reach down to put the garment over the sound foot. Many patients are unable to maintain sitting balance whilst moving the sound foot off the ground. These patients should keep the sound heel on the ground while putting garments over the sound toes, then keep the sound toes on the ground while pulling the garment round the sound heel. Such patients should then stand up, achieve standing balance, and pull up garments into their final position. If appropriate, the patient may weight bear through his/her affected upper limb when standing to pull up garments. Great care needs to be taken if doing this not to cause damage to the wrist. Patients should be taught to tie shoelaces one-handed as soon as possible.

To remove all lower garments:

The patient should lower all garments while standing, and remove them the opposite way to putting them on.

Commonly encountered problems in dressing include:

(a) bras: these can be changed to front opening or hooked up and put on like a jumper. Alternatively, looser support/sports bras can be used;
(b) not being able to reach round the back to put the arm in a sleeve. This may be done up and put on like a jumper over the head;
(c) not being able to do up a trouser top. This may be adapted with Velcro fastenings;
(d) shoe laces: spring lacers may be used or laces may be laced one-handed as in Figures 3.1 and 3.2.

To lace shoe: **Knot one end of the lace and thread through shoe as shown in the diagram below**

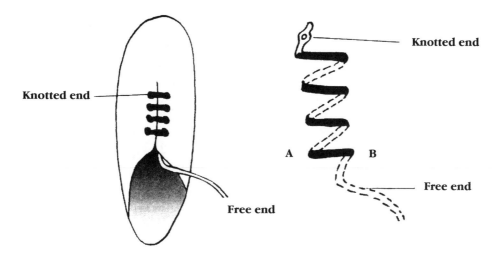

To tie shoe: **Loop free end of lace over AB.**

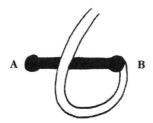

Make a second loop with free end of lace, pass it under AB and through first loop

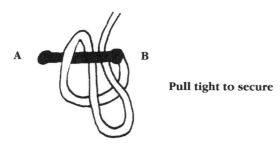

Pull tight to secure

Figure 3.1 Instructions for tying shoelaces one-handed.

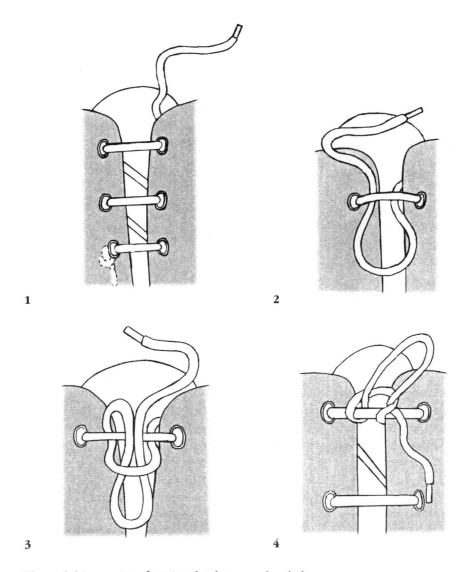

1   2   3   4

Figure 3.2 Instructions for tying shoelaces one-handed.

Feeding

Most patients will be able to feed themselves using one hand, but care should be taken to prevent choking. Advice may need to be obtained from a speech and language therapist and/or dietitian.

Below is a suggested technique for mealtimes:

• The patient should sit in a chair with arms (preferably), or in a wheelchair, at a table for meals. If a wheelchair has to be used, extra attention needs to be given to the positioning of the patient.

- He/she should be positioned close to the table, sitting upright, which may require having a pillow behind his/her back to support him/her.
- His/her feet should be flat on the floor with hips, knees and ankles at 90 degrees.
- Ideally he/she should have his/her affected arm out straight in front of him/her across the table, keeping the affected shoulder protracted. However, this is not always practical and if the trunk is well positioned, the affected arm may be placed on the affected knee to maintain inhibition of the stroke pattern.

Common problems with feeding include:

(a) inability to cut food: this may be helped by use of a rocker knife and non-slip mat under the plate;
(b food moving off the plate: advise use of a plate guard or plate with a lip;
(c) weak grip in recovering hand: use enlarged grips on cutlery;
(d) difficulty seeing all of food on plate owing to hemianopia: teach patient to rotate plate and scan.

Instrumental Activities

Household tasks need to be approached with an understanding of the patient's needs and wants. Position the task and patient to facilitate ease of reach and balance. When in a wheelchair the use of a tray fixed in front allows the patient to transport items and work at a good height.

As the patient progresses, there is a tendency to provide the pelvis with extra stability from the shoulder girdle by retracting and depressing the scapula; this can be discouraged by the use of a perching stool. Perch sitting allows greater freedom of movement in the upper limb and facilitates easier reach in the affected side.

Kitchen activities

A suggested technique for kitchen activities is outlined below:

- This could include tasks such as making a hot drink, cooking snacks or meals, baking, handwashing or ironing.
- The patient could carry out these activities from a wheelchair, chair, perching stool or in a standing position.
- Particular emphasis should be placed on the movements used to carry out these tasks, to prevent abnormal increases in tone on the affected side. For example, a patient standing unsupported and trying to pour boiling water from a kettle may use excess effort and, combined with the anxiety

caused by the risk of scalding or falling, is likely to have an abnormal increase in tone in the affected side.
- The patient should be taught to consider the position and safety of the affected upper limb and an awareness of hazards, e.g. when using hot liquids, cookers or irons. The effect anxiety has on increasing tone should also be remembered in all kitchen activities.

There are many pieces of equipment to assist with meal preparation and the patient will need advice on those most suitable for his/her needs. The following are suggestions:

(a) stabilizing objects: advise use of non-slip mats, pan holders on the stove, spike boards, buttering boards etc.;
(b) cutting objects: use of food processors, spiked chopping boards, adapted knives, may be helpful;
(c) opening items: suggest electric can openers, mounted jar openers, belli-clamps;
(d) carrying items: advise use of a trolley or one-handed tray.

Cleaning and laundry

Most patients will initially tackle the tasks from a wheelchair, but as they improve, these tasks provide the therapist with a wealth of opportunities to encourage mobility, balance, upper limb recovery, hand coordination and dexterity.

Items that may assist with these activities include:

(a) long-handled tools to facilitate ease of reach;
(b) an 'easy-reach' to enable items to be picked up from the floor;
(c) trolleys to help with moving items around;
(d) perching stools, to assist with static standing tasks such as washing up and ironing, and an adjustable height ironing board.

Household repairs

Unless the patient makes a significant recovery these tasks are often left to outside agencies. Even so, if the patient is particularly interested in DIY there are a number of tasks that can facilitate recovery of the hemiplegic side.

These include:

(a) sanding, using affected hand, which encourages active control around the shoulder, elbow and gross grip;
(b) use of hand tools with care, e.g. a light hammer, promotes rhythmic control of movement.

NB:*These tasks must be carefully monitored to inhibit associated reactions, prevent undue increases in tone and to check for undesirable compensation by other muscles.*

There are a number of gadgets that are available to help stabilize work, but the exact needs will have to be individually assessed.

Remedial Activities

In the management of physical problems following stroke, remedial activities offer the patient movement experience in a controlled environment. The therapist positions the task to gain specific movements, often related to regaining upper limb function. Unless the patient has an interest in playing board games these will need to be used with care and explanation. They do offer the patient repeated exposure to specific movement patterns required for functional tasks that would be difficult to gain by the use of ADL tasks alone.

Principles of management

(a) Tasks should be positioned to achieve a specific movement/movement sequence, e.g. positioned to encourage weight transference to the affected side, or to encourage forward flexion to help facilitate standing.
(b) Each task should demand a higher cognitive function, to prevent attention being exclusively focused on the movement. This allows the patient to learn how to multitask information, e.g. walking and turning the head at the same time to cross the road.
(c) The patient should understand why the therapist has chosen a task.
(d) Each activity should be able to be related to a functional task, e.g. reaching forward and up for a game may relate to reaching into a cupboard.

Summary

The therapist plays a key role in the initial stages of recovery from a stroke. The therapist can help the patient gain independence and dignity while at the time setting the foundation for recovery and long-term functional gains. The therapist needs to understand the patient in the context of his/her daily life and plan therapy that helps the patient see a realistic future, regardless of any remaining deficits.

Chapter 4
Management of
Cognitive/Perceptual Deficits

Cognition

Classification

Lezak (1995) divided cognition into four aspects, as in computer operations:

* *Input*:
    - receptive functions: ability to select, acquire, classify and integrate information,
      i.e. sensation, perception, attention, concentration.
* *Storage*:
    - memory and learning: ability to store and retrieve information,
      i.e. verbal and visual memory, registration, short-term memory, immediate memory, long-term memory, remote memory.
* *Processing*:
    - thinking: ability to mentally organize and reorganize information,
      i.e. reasoning, judgement, executive functioning.
* *Output*:
    - expressive functions: means through which information is communicated or acted upon,
      i.e. apraxia, aphasia.

Malia and Brannagan (1997), however, classify cognition into the following five aspects:
* *Attention*:
    - focused;
    - sustained;
    - selective;
    - alternating;
    - divided.
* *Visual Processing*:
    (i) Visual cognition:

- spatial problem;
- alexia;
- figure–ground;
- position in space;
- constructional problem;
- contextual clues to gain meaning for an image.

(ii) Visual memory

(iii) Pattern recognition:
- colour;
- shape;
- contour;
- texture;
- detail.

(iv) Scanning

(v) Visual attention

(vi) Oculomotor skills:
- visual field;
- visual acuity.

- *Memory*:

(i) Sensory memory:
- attending.

(ii) Short-term (waking) memory
- encoding.

(iii) Long-term (semantic) memory
- storage;
- retrieval.

- *Information Processing*:
- classification of received information;
- memory;
- organizational skills:

i.e. separating;
  closure;
  combining;
  sorting;
  ranking;
  sequencing;
  categorizing;
  grouping.

- *Executive Functions*:
- self-awareness;
- goal setting;
- self-initiation;
- self-inhibition;

- planning;
- self-monitoring and self-evaluation;
- flexible problem solving.

Assessment of Cognition

There many standardized cognitive assessments available, some of which are available from the Thames Valley Test Company, NFER-Nelson and Psychological Corporation. Courses are available from the Thames Valley Test Company, NFER-Nelson and the College of Occupational Therapists' 'Objective and standardized assessments course', which ensure occupational therapists get the full benefit of using these assessments.

These may include assessments such as:

- Attention – Test of Everyday Attention (TEA) (Robertson et al., 1994).
- Cognition – Middlesex Elderly Assessment of Mental State (MEAMS) (Golding, 1989).
- Memory – Wechsler Memory Scale (Wechsler, 1987);
  - Recognition Memory Test (Warrington, 1984);
  - Rivermead Behavioural Memory Test (RBMT) (Wilson et al., 1985);
  - Salford Objective Recognition Test (SORT) (Burgess et al., 1994);
  - Subjective Memory Questionnaire (Bennett-Levy and Powell, 1980).
- Reasoning – Coloured Progressive Matrices (Raven, 1958);
  - Cognitive Estimates (Shallice and Evans, 1978);
  - Word Fluency (Benton and Hamsher, 1989);
  - Modified Card Sorting Test (Nelson, 1976).
- Perception – Chessington Occupational Therapy Neurological Assessment Battery (COTNAB) (Tyerman et al., 1986);
  - Loewenstein Occupational Therapy Cognitive Assessment (LOTCA) (Itzkovich et al., 1993);
  - Rey figure copying test (Rey, 1959);
  - Rivermead Behavioural Inattention Test (BIT) (Wilson et al., 1987)
  - Rivermead Perceptual Assessment Battery (RPAB) (Whiting et al., 1985; Lincoln and Edmans, 1989);
  - Visual Object & Spatial Perception Battery (VOSP) (Warrington and James, 1991).
    (see section on perception also)
- Apraxia – Kertesz Apraxia Test (Kertesz and Ferro, 1984).
  (see section on dyspraxia also)
- Executive functions – Hayling and Brixton Tests (Burgess and Shallice, 1997);
  - Behavioural Assessment of Dysexecutive Syndrome (BADS) (Wilson et al., 1996).

Treatment of Cognitive Deficits

Malia and Brannagan (1997) suggest treatment as a threefold approach:

1. *Skills Training*: concentrating on the component cognitive skills under-lying all function.
2. *Strategy Training*: focusing on teaching compensation approaches, e.g. goal planning, task analysis, demonstration .
3. *Functional Skills Training*: using specifically relevant activities, i.e. everyday tasks.

Specific activities that could be used in the treatment of cognitive problems include:

- *Attention*
  - computer games.
- *Memory*
  - external aids:
    notebooks;
    calendars;
    diaries;
    cooking timers/alarm clock;
    audio cassette;
    signposts/notices/labels;
    knots in hankies;
    timetable;
    computer-assisted technology.
- Patients need to be trained to use them.
- Specific aids are needed for specific tasks.
- Patients initially need supervision in their use.
- Most likely strategy to be effective.
  - internal aids (mnemonics):
    visual
    - visual imagery (useful for names);
    - mental retracing;
    - motor coding;
    - pictorial instructions;
    verbal
    - PQRST (preview, question, read, state, test);
    - rhymes;
    - first letter cueing.
- Mnemonics have to be taught in relation to a specific practical task.
- Some strategies can only be applied to a few tasks to avoid confusion.
- Can be discrepancies between visual and verbal memory.
- Can be taught in groups.

- May help patient to cope with problem but will not affect underlying deficit.
- *Reasoning*
  - problem-solving strategies may help but it depends on patient's awareness of problem.

Perceptual Deficits

Siev and Freishtat (1976) describe three main deficit areas:

1. body image and scheme;
2. spatial relations;
3. agnosia.

- *Body image deficit* is the lack of visual and mental image of one's body. This relates to the feelings and thoughts of the body, rather than the physical structure.
- *Body scheme deficit* is the difficulty in perceiving the position of the body and the relationship of body parts. This is needed in order to know what, where and how to move oneself.
  - *Somatognosia* is the lack of awareness of the body structure and relationships, causing the patient to confuse sides of the body and body parts.
  - *Unilateral neglect* is the neglect of the affected side of the body or the environment.
  - *Anosognosia* is the lack of recognition of the presence or severity of the paralysis, or complete denial of the illness.
  - *Right/left discrimination deficit* is the difficulty in understanding the concept of right and left.
  - *Finger agnosia* is the difficulty in knowing which finger is touched when there is no sensory loss, causing dexterity problems.

- *Spatial relations deficit* is the difficulty in perceiving the position of two or more objects in relation to oneself or each other, e.g. difficulty putting food onto a spoon and then into the mouth or difficulty putting a teapot lid on a teapot.
  - *Figure–ground deficit* is the difficulty in distinguishing the foreground from the background, e.g. difficulty finding a brush in a cluttered drawer or a white shirt on a white sheet.
  - *Form constancy deficit* is the difficulty in attending to subtle variations in form, e.g. difficulty differentiating between a water jug and flower vase.
  - *Position in space deficit* is the difficulty in understanding the concepts of in/out, front/behind, up/down etc., e.g. difficulty finding a cup behind a kettle.
  - *Topographical disorientation* is the difficulty in understanding and

remembering relationships of places to one another, e.g. difficulty in finding one's way.

- *Depth and distance deficit* is the difficulty in judging depth and distance, e.g. difficulty navigating stairs and barriers such as walls or doorways or difficulty knowing when a glass is full when filling it with water.
- *Agnosia* is the lack of recognition of familiar objects perceived by the senses, i.e. visual, tactile, proprioceptive, auditory or body scheme.
  - *Visual object agnosia* is the difficulty in recognizing objects although visual acuity and visual fields are intact, e.g. a patient may fail to recognize relatives or possessions.
  - *Simultanognosia* is the difficulty in absorbing more than one aspect of a whole picture, e.g. a patient may be able to pick out a single letter but be unable to read a complete word.
  - *Prosopagnosia* is the difficulty in recognizing differences in faces.
  - *Colour agnosia* is the difficulty in recognizing colours.
  - *Metamorphopsia* is the difficulty in realizing the actual size of an object.
  - *Visual spatial agnosia* is the difficulty in perceiving spatial relationships between objects or between objects and self, independently of visual object agnosia.
  - *Tactile agnosia* (also called astereognosis) is the difficulty in recognizing objects by handling, although tactile, thermal and proprioceptive functions are intact.
  - *Auditory agnosia* is the difficulty in recognizing differences in sounds, including both word and non-word sounds, e.g. a patient may be unable to differentiate between the sound of a car engine running and the sound of a vacuum cleaner.
  - *Apractognosia* is a term given for a collection of deficits i.e., body scheme, spatial relations, apraxia and agnosia.

Analysis of Perceptual Assessment Results

When analysing the results of a perceptual assessment, it is important to consider the effect of other abilities which may affect perceptual performance, as well as the actual perceptual assessment scores, such as:

- use of the non-dominant hand;
- language;
- comprehension;
- concentration and attention;
- initiation;
- dyspraxia;
- reasoning;
- memory;

- depression;
- anxiety;
- hemianopia or diplopia;
- eyesight;
- overall affect of inattention.

When the analysis has been made, the results should be explained to the patient, i.e.:
- which subtests they had problems with;
- what the perceptual problem is called;
- how that perceptual problem may affect them in everyday life;
- what treatment can be offered.

The results should also be explained to all staff involved with that patient and to the patient's relatives.

Treatment of Perceptual Deficits

There are several approaches to the treatment of perceptual deficits, described by Zoltan in her book *Vision, Perception and Cognition* (1996) and by Zoltan et al. in their book *The Adult Stroke Patient* (1986).

Bottom-up approaches (remedial treatment) assume that the patient will be able to generalize this treatment to activities of daily living, e.g.:

- transfer of training;
- sensory integration;
- neurodevelopmental;
- Affolter.

Top-down approaches (adaptive treatment) promote adaptation of and to the environment to capitalize on the patient's abilities, e.g.:

- occupational performance;
- functional;
- dynamic interactional.

Transfer of training approach

The basic assumption of this approach is that practice on a particular perceptual task will affect the patient's performance on similar perceptual tasks. For example, a patient with difficulty dressing due to a spatial relations deficit may practice cube-copying tasks, in the hope that he/she improves functionally in areas involving spatial relations, such as dressing.

Sensory integration approach

This approach is based on the work of Ayres (1980) for use when treating children with perceptual, cognitive or behavioural problems. The underlying assumption is that sensory integration is the organization of sensation for use. Sensory integration converts our initial sensations into meaningful perceptions and sensory integration occurs during an adaptive response.

Neurodevelopmental approach

The emphasis in this approach is on inhibiting abnormal reflex mechanisms and facilitating normal movement. Tactile and kinesthetic stimulation through handling and movement is provided to encourage contact between the individual and the environment. The redevelopment of normal postural movement makes possible redevelopment of the normal body scheme, leading to improved perceptual and visual discrimination skills. The use of the 'forced use' technique can change the functional capacity of the patient and the patient must learn through functional activities. Motor learning is affected by movement organization, environmental factors and cognitive processing. Movement analysis should include all systems that affect movement.

Affolter approach

This approach assumes that the tactile-kinesthetic system is key to problem solving and that effective problem solving leads to learning and independence. In order to learn, the patient must experience learning situations and interact with the environment. Treatment is process-orientated and focuses on the input.

Occupational performance

The assumption is that the individual is an open system that exists through the interaction between the individual and the environment. This relationship is a performance transaction and there are three levels of occupational performance: activities, tasks and roles. Activities require certain sensorimotor, cognitive, perceptual, emotional and social abilities. An individual must be able to do the tasks that make up a role in order to satisfactorily engage in a life role and achieve competence.

Functional approach

The patient is made aware of his/her problems and taught to compensate for them, or the environment or task is adapted to maximize function. It is the repetitive practice of particular tasks, usually ADL tasks, which will make the patient more independent in meeting his/her basic needs. The emphasis is on treating the symptom rather than the cause of the problem. For example, a patient with a spatial relations deficit who has difficulty dressing may practise dressing until he/she can dress him/herself, but he will still have the underlying spatial relations deficit.

Dynamic interactional approach

In this approach, the patient is made aware of his/her problems and taught to compensate for them, or the environment or task is adapted to maximize function. Patient performance is analysed by examining the underlying conditions and processing strategies that change performance. Evaluation and treatment are carried out in a variety of situations or contexts (multi-context). Multi-context learning promotes generalization and use of information and strategies across task situations.

Perceptual Treatment Plan

1. Assess perceptual and ADL abilities using standardized assessments.
2. Analyse results and consider the effects of:
   – comprehension;
   – concentration;
   – reasoning;
   – initiation;
   – memory;
   – anxiety;
   – depression;
   – dyspraxia;
   – hemianopia/eyesight;
   – inattention.
3. Explain to the patient, relatives and all staff involved the patient's specific perceptual problems and the likely effects of these in everyday life.
4. Choose the treatment approach to be used.
5. Decide which treatment strategies to use.
6. Relate the treatment to the patient's needs.
7. Remember that not everyone likes games and puzzles.
8. Remember that we all learn in different ways.
9. Give mental stimulation.
10. Reassess perceptual and ADL abilities.

General Perceptual Treatment Strategies

1. Consider the complexity of the task that the patient is doing, i.e. start with simple tasks and gradually build up to more complicated tasks (Hecaen and Assal, 1970).
2. Consider using demonstration, imitation or gesture, to facilitate the patient during activities.

3. Consider whether to use verbal or written instructions.
4. Remember that one of the accepted elements of learning is repetition and practice.
5. Reinforce positive behaviours rather than negative ones.
6. Give general mental stimulation to encourage active participation by the patient.
7. Facilitate the patient by staging components, i.e. breaking down tasks into stages and encouraging the patient to complete one stage at a time.
8. Facilitate the patient by giving verbal or physical cues and prompting.
9. Try to establish set patterns and routines for carrying out each activity, i.e. be systematic.
10. Ensure consistency in approach and method of treatment by the whole team.

Specific Perceptual Treatment Strategies

The two most commonly used approaches to the treatment of perceptual problems, which are suitable for use with adult brain-damaged patients, are the transfer of training and functional approaches. Specific strategies for specific perceptual problems and examples of treatment using these two approaches are given below.

Body image and body scheme

Aim: To increase the patient's awareness of the relationship of parts of the body and how they are needed in order to carry out activities.

Strategies:

1. Encourage the patient to verbalize parts of his/her body during functional activities or when using appropriate puzzle-type activities (Anderson and Choy, 1970).
2. Encourage the patient to identify parts of the body on him/herself or on the therapist to improve his/her recognition of parts of his/her body (Anderson and Choy, 1970).
3. Encourage the patient to verbalize the position of parts of his/her body, to improve his/her body awareness (Anderson and Choy, 1970).

Transfer of training activities:

- assembling manikin puzzles of a man, woman or a face;
- drawing and naming parts of a body, stick man or a face;
- using clothes cards to identify where they fit on a body.

Functional activities:

- washing: using instructions such as wash your arm, face or chest, touch or name parts of the body, or using a mirror during cleaning teeth or combing hair;

- dressing: using instructions such as put your left arm into the sleeve, push clothes over your right shoulder, put your watch on your right wrist;
- transfers: using instructions such as hold your wrist.

Unilateral neglect

Aim: To make the patient aware of both sides of the environment.

Strategies:

1. Place objects to be used during the activity initially in the midline and graduate by moving the objects further to the patient's affected side (Burt, 1970).
2. Encourage staff to approach the patient from the patient's affected side (Burt, 1970).
3. Place the stimulus on the patient's affected side, e.g. wash kit/clothes/tapping the table (Burt, 1970).
4. Prompt and encourage the patient to look to his/her affected side (Burt, 1970).
5. Use activities that cross the patient's midline.
6. Emphasize the patient's affected side during activities (Burt, 1970).
7. Adapt the environment to make tasks easier for the patient, e.g. positioning objects so the patient is aware of where the object is (Pigott and Brickett, 1966).
8. Use environmental landmarks, e.g. edge of table/carpet/window, red line on affected side of task (Pigott and Brickett, 1966; Diller, 1981). The patient is taught to look to his/her affected side to locate the edge of furniture etc., in order to orientate the patient to that side and to work back to the midline to find the objects or task in hand.

Transfer of training activities:

- drawing/copying a house, clock etc.;
- cancellation tasks (Diller, 1981), maze or word search puzzles;
- using a red line on the affected side as a stimulus (Diller 1981);
- using computer games with a touch screen (Robertson et al., 1988);
- using a visual field scanner (similar to Diller's 'scanning machine') (Diller and Weinberg, 1977);
- any wide-angled games that require the patient to scan the visual field, e.g. large-sized dominoes.

Functional activities:

- washing: following general strategies, e.g. putting objects to the affected side of the wash bowl or washing the affected arm;
- dressing: crossing legs when dressing the lower half of the body, putting clothes or check list on the affected side, putting tape round sleeve hole of affected arm or dressing the affected arm first;
- grooming: using a mirror and ensuring the patient shaves both sides of his face;
- eating: encouraging the patient to turn the plate round to find his/her food;
- transfers: moving towards a chair or similar on the affected side of the patient;
- gardening/kitchen tasks: tasks involving crossing the midline or putting items on the affected side of the patient.
- reading a paragraph aloud or copying a paragraph.

Spatial relations

Aim: To make the patient aware of the relationship of objects to objects or self, to identify foreground from background, position in space, and depth and distance.

Strategies:

1. Encourage the patient to use a variable numbers of objects in a task, i.e. start with a few items and build up to having lots of items around in a cluttered surrounding (Hecaen and Assal, 1970).
2. Encourage the patient to find items from a contrasting or similar background (Taylor, 1969).
3. Encourage the patient to pick out objects in the foreground from the background.
4. Encourage the patient to trace around outlines of objects, pictures etc., to facilitate identifying objects and positions.
5. Encourage the patient to identify overlapping figures or items.
6. Encourage the patient to verbalize the relationships of items to him/herself or items to each other, during functional and transfer of training tasks.
7. Consider the terms used in verbal instructions, e.g. in/out, front/behind (Taylor, 1969).
8. Try to relate the terms used to other objects, e.g. move towards the chair or person.
9. Encourage the patient to verbalize the recognition of shapes and positions in 2D and 3D situations.
10. Encourage the patient to verbalize the recognition of the depth and distance of objects etc.

Transfer of training activities:

- varieties of domino-type games, e.g. spot on, heads and tails, symmetry or jigsaw dominoes, connect or triominoes;
- what's in the square puzzle;
- cards to make two-dimensional block-design-type patterns (Wechsler, 1955);
- three-dimensional block-design tasks (Wechsler, 1955);
- cube or three-dimensional copying tasks (Anderson and Choy, 1970);
- geometrix puzzle.

Functional activities:

- washing: putting soap on contrasting colour cloth and progressing to using white soap on a white cloth or sink, identifying the relationship of objects, e.g. soap to soap dish, flannel to water, toothbrush to toothpaste;
- dressing: finding clothes in a cluttered drawer or in a pile on the bed, using a contrasting coloured background, arranging clothes so sleeve hole is visible or outlining sleeve hole with red tape or marking back of clothes (Burt, 1970);
- kitchen tasks: putting teabags into a teapot, identifying the relationship of objects needed for the task, filling the kettle, teapot etc., finding objects in cluttered surroundings;
- mealtimes: facilitating the awareness of the relationship of food to cutlery, cutlery to mouth and cutlery to plate.
- gardening: facilitating the awareness of relationship of plants, pots and compost;
- stairs: facilitating the awareness of relationship of stairs to feet, and depth and distance of stairs.

Agnosia and form constancy

Aim: To improve ability to distinguish differences in form, colour, etc.

Strategies:

1. Encourage the patient to recognize differences and similarities between items.
2. Start with items that are very different and graduate to items that are very similar, with subtle variations, e.g. shapes, sizes, colours.
3. Encourage the patient to verbalize differences, i.e. naming objects and differences between objects.

Transfer of training activities:

- variety of domino-type games, e.g. matching numbers, colours, shapes, pictures, symmetrical and reversed shapes etc.;

- colour- and shape-matching blocks;
- inset-placing games involving recognition of similarities and differences;
- challenge games involving recognition of similarities and differences;
- what's in the square puzzle involving recognition of similarities and differences;
- lookalikes games involving recognition of similarities and differences.

Functional activities:

Recognition in everyday situations of objects, colours, sizes and subtle variations in form/colour, e.g. tins, fruits, vegetables, plates and saucers etc., according to which agnosia the patient has, during:

- washing;
- dressing;
- bathing;
- kitchen tasks;
- shopping;
- gardening.

Chapter 5
Resettlement

Mood

Anxiety and depression are likely to make rehabilitation difficult for patients as they may have decreased motivation to participate in assessments and treatment due to being preoccupied with their worries and thoughts. DeSouza (1983) also noted that one of the major factors affecting the success of stroke rehabilitation was the patient's own determination and motivation to improve functionally. The nature of depression is that depressed patients are likely to have a decreased ability for motivation. This finding was supported by Zigmond and Snaith (1983), who suggested that patients may find that symptoms of their illness distress them to such an extent as to lead to a poor response to treatment. Ebrahim et al. (1987) also demonstrated that mood disturbance at six months post-stroke was strongly associated with functional ability, limb weakness and with longer hospital stay. This suggests that slow recovery and institutionalization may be responsible for mood disturbances.

Similarly, Robinson et al. (1983) found that in 103 patients, the severity of impairment in functional activities (ADL) and intellectual function was significantly correlated with the severity of post-stroke depression early after stroke. Sixty-one of the patients in their study were reassessed after six months and were found to have made a significant improvement in functional impairment (Robinson et al., 1984). However, the depressed patients remained more impaired that the non-depressed patients.

A further study by Sinyor et al. (1986) also indicated that depression was common after stroke. They demonstrated that depression was associated with the level of functional impairment in 64 depressed stroke patients early after stroke and suggested that it may cause a negative impact on the rehabilitation process and outcome. They followed up 25 of these patients, six months after discharge, and still found a significant correlation between depression and functional status.

All these studies (Robinson et al., 1984; Sinyor et al., 1986; Ebrahim et al., 1987) used standardized assessments for mood and functional ability but the Robinson et al. and Sinyor et al. studies had small numbers of patients.

Thus the effect of any of these impairments has been shown to be associated with functional ability, highlighting the complexity and trauma of stroke. It is therefore important to consider the effect of these impairments, the 'invisible consequences of stroke', when treating any patient following stroke.

Depression

The symptoms of depression may include:

- negative thoughts;
- irrational beliefs;
- distortion of reality;
- self-blame;
- all-or-nothing attitude;
- low mood;
- poor appetite and weight loss;
- increased appetite and weight gain;
- disturbed sleep;
- activity alters -> lethargic or agitated;
- loss of interest and pleasure;
- poor concentration;
- indecision.

Assessments that may be used include:

(a) Hospital Anxiety & Depression Scale (Zigmond and Snaith, 1983);
(b) Wakefield Depression Inventory (Snaith et al., 1971);
(c) Geriatric Depression Scale (Agrell and Dehlin, 1989);
(d) General Health Questionnaire (Goldberg and Hiller, 1979).

Treatment may involve counselling, antidepressants or psychological treatment. Behavioural treatment could include reinforcing activity, activity scheduling, feedback of progress, experiencing success or pleasant events. Long-term therapy from a psychologist or psychiatrist may be required for some patients. This will depend on the severity of the depression and the patient's ability to cope with the depression. Occasionally patients may become so depressed that they feel suicidal, in which case medical advice should be sought. Some patients may turn to spirituality to assist them in coping with the new life-style forced upon them.

Anxiety

Patients may have anxieties relating to their stroke, e.g. fear of having another stroke, fear of epilepsy, fear regarding their future in terms of home, social, sex or employment contexts.

The Hospital Anxiety & Depression Scale (Zigmond and Snaith, 1983) may be used for assessment.

Treatment may include counselling, tranquillizers or psychological treatment.

Lability (now often called 'emotionalism')

Patients may have difficulty in controlling their emotions, such that they cry or laugh as a result of any alteration in emotions, which can be very distressing for them.

The most effective way to treat this lability is to ignore it, as attention to the problem invariably makes it worse. The patient should be given reassurance instead. Distraction techniques are sometimes effective.

Fatigue (Carr and Shepherd, 1987; Laidler 1994)

Fatigue is part of any illness or traumatic event and can affect the individual physically, mentally, emotionally, or as a mixture of all three. It is usually expected and apparent in the acute stage following stroke, but can also appear as a persistent problem long after discharge from hospital.

In the initial stages following stroke, the systems of the body are working to promote recovery, and the patient has to make a great deal of effort – for example in working on sitting or concentrating on a task. Some degree of exhaustion is inevitable, and therapists should be aware that many patients feel they are being worked too hard and that we do not understand their situation.

After discharge, the person feels that because he/she is 'better', he/she should manage as before, but those tasks which were once easy now require continuing effort to perform, be they getting dressed, holding a conversation or reading a book.

Therapists expect patients to get fatigued, and are encouraged not to overtire them as this can lead to increased tone, poor performance, reduced motivation and so on. However, the patient who appears fatigued may not actually be tired following effort. Patients should be able to tolerate periods of reasonably challenging activity and the fatigue that accompanies such activity should easily respond to a period of rest. Fatigue within normal limits does not affect learning, although it may temporarily affect performance. First, we should look at the background reasons as to why the patient may be complaining about or showing signs of fatigue, and then address the issues involved. It may be that he/she is not sleeping well at night, is not able to wake in the day because of medication, is anxious or depressed, has an infection or other pathological condition, is poorly nourished or suffering from boredom. This last may well be the most important cause of fatigue!

The patient should not have to use a huge amount of physical effort – the effort should be on the part of the therapist, with relaxed reciprocation from the patient. Treatment should involve successful activity, be challenging but not impossible and not cause stress. Working with therapists involves both physical and mental effort on the patient's part and it can be more effective to change the task than stop and rest when a patient appears tired. Carr and Shepherd report studies in normal subjects that show muscle work performed after a diverting activity was greater than that performed after a rest – and they report one study with a small group of stroke patients that appeared to support this. As an alternative to activity or rest, suitable relaxation techniques can be taught to the patient.

Once discharged from hospital, it can be helpful for the person to understand the possible causes of his/her tiredness, and discuss strategies for coping with it. These would involve keeping active and returning to or developing interests, using energy wisely, dealing with concerns and depression.

Therapists should be aware of the patient's sense of fatigue, explain their understanding of it, and why it may appear that they are ignoring it. By providing a varied and challenging programme, they will assist the patient in handling fatigue.

Resuming Sexual Activity (Edmans, 1998)

The rehabilitation of stroke patients is constantly improving, there are many new techniques and ideas. However, one area often neglected is patients returning to their normal sexual activity. Generally, this is not routinely discussed with patients as part of their rehabilitation, although for many it plays an important role in their life.

There is some information in a few stroke books, but this is not always readily available to the patient and his/her partner and the information is not always applicable to their specific needs. Lynch and Grisogono (1991) reported that if patients had a sexual relationship prior to their stroke, there was no reason not to continue post-stroke. They also stated that the sensation of the genital organs is normally unaffected after a stroke and sexual intercourse is not dangerous for the patient's blood pressure. This has been backed up by Mulley (1985), Youngson (1987) and Wade (1988), who have also stated that sexual intercourse is quite safe after stroke. Mulley suggested that sexual enjoyment may be reduced as a result of motor or sensory impairment or due to a general breakdown of marriage or relationships, which may occur after any disabling illness. A study of aphasic patients by Kinsella and Duffy (1979) found that only 17% of couples continued sexual intercourse and then usually at diminished frequency. Grieve (1995) reported patients' physical problems as being due to catheters, speech, vision, hearing, neglect, weakness, spasticity, sensibility, dressing and pain difficulties, along with psychological problems of identity, dependency, self-esteem and principles of behaviour.

After a stroke, generally both patients and partners want to know whether resuming sexual activity will cause another stroke or epileptic fit, and do not know who to discuss the subject with.

In a recent study by Edmans (1998), patients and partners reported the following reasons as to why their sexual life had deteriorated since the stroke: lack of interest or motivation on the part of one or both of the couple, physical incapacity of the patient, difficulty getting in a comfortable position for both of the couple, difficulty getting their partner aroused and difficulties due to sensory deficits on the patient's affected side.

Patients and partners reported that they would have liked to receive information on why problems occurred in resuming sexual activity after a stroke and how long they were likely to last. Some also reported that they would have liked there to be more opportunity to discuss their fears and problems, especially after discharge from hospital.

The Stroke Association has now produced a leaflet, entitled *Sex after Stroke Illness*, which includes the main points that were identified by patients and partners. This leaflet should be made available to all stroke patients and their partners.

Sexual activity is a subject which is important to both patients and partners, and should be included in stroke rehabilitation. However, despite this, it is still not clear cut whose role should encompass this or whether it should be part of the role of all staff involved in the rehabilitation of stroke patients. Patients and partners should have the opportunity to choose who they wish to undertake this role.

There is also no set time when and how this subject should be introduced, suggesting that information and advice should perhaps be made more readily available to patients and partners throughout their stay in hospital. Patients and partners need to know that returning to their normal sexual activity is considered routinely as an aspect of stroke rehabilitation. They also need to know that there is the opportunity to discuss their sexual activity either alone or as a couple, at a time that is appropriate to their needs.

Patients can also get support and advice from the Association for the Sexual and Personal Relationships of the Disabled (SPOD), 286 Camden Road, London N7 0BJ.

Leisure Rehabilitation

It is known that participation in leisure decreases after stroke (Labi et al., 1980; Sjogren, 1982; Drummond 1990). The significance of this reduction lies in the fact that previous studies have shown that satisfactory leisure is related to life satisfaction (Mancini, 1978; Allen & Beattie, 1984; Sneegas, 1986). Consequently such a decrease in leisure activity may reflect a decrease in quality of life.

There is a growing feeling that not enough is done to enable patients who have had a stroke to resume former hobbies or acquire new interests. Greveson and James (1991), reporting on the results of a study into long-term outcome after stroke, concluded that:

> Little help or advice had been given to patients to participate in leisure interests such as gardening, painting, or sewing, and patients thought that this could have appreciably improved their quality of life.

In Nottingham, work has been conducted on providing programmes of leisure rehabilitation after stroke (Drummond and Walker, 1995; Parker et al., 1999). Below are some practical tips from the experiences of occupational therapists, which may help those considering similar projects with their patients:

- It may be best to ask patients what they did in their free time, rather than using the word 'leisure'. Many people, particularly the elderly, do not understand the word and equate it with laziness (which is emphatically to be denied!).
- Decide on a definition of leisure. Consider, for example, if individuals report that they spend their leisure time ironing and dusting – is that acceptable to you? The definition used by us was: 'activity chosen primarily for its own sake after the practical necessities of life have been attended to' (Drummond, 1990) (i.e. this definition does not include household chores, no matter how enjoyable the individual reports them to be!).
- Keep a written record of what patients did before their stroke. This will enable you to identify areas of interest and plan a programme. Responses are usually more comprehensive when a checklist (such as the Nottingham Leisure Questionnaire – Drummond and Walker, 1994) is used than when an open question about interests is asked.
- Discuss a possible programme with the patient. Some people are happy to resume former hobbies at a slower pace; others prefer to try something completely new so that they are not reminded of their disability.
- Look at common themes from the checklist, which may help you to suggest new hobbies. For example, does someone like solitary activities? Outdoor pursuits? Competitive interests?
- Do not overlook, in favour of the more exciting, eye-catching interests, the most common everyday activities, such as:
  - watching TV/videos;
  - radio/music;

- reading newspapers, magazines and books;
- gardening;
- baking;
- going for a walk;
- visiting the pub.

- Consider the most obvious limitations to carrying out hobbies. For example, assess the need for new spectacles or a new hearing aid before assessing problems with hand function and balance.
- Do not overlook patients who have made a good physical recovery from their stroke. Previous studies (e.g. Labi et al., 1980) have shown that these patients often also have reduced leisure performance.
- Link up patients with similar hobbies and interests.
- Encourage help and support from family and friends. Tap into local resources such as voluntary agencies for additional help.
- Keep a box file of local resources and facilities, such as:
  - local clubs;
  - Dial-A-Ride services;
  - travel agencies specializing in holiday accommodation for the disabled;
  - any special local facilities (swimming sessions for the disabled, fishing sites for disabled fishermen, local riding-for-the-disabled stables).
- Contact national organizations for local contacts if you are unable to access facilities yourself.
- Browse through specialist equipment catalogues which may give you more ideas for hobbies. Remember that some equipment may be bought cheaper in larger stores than from specialist firms.
- Ask for donations of books, jigsaws, board games etc. and keep a store for lending out equipment.
- Funding! Consider specific charities and local groups such as the Hospital League of Friends, and Rotary Clubs for specialist one-off items for individuals. Encourage the patient's family to consider buying expensive items, such as gardening equipment, as birthday or Christmas presents.
- Be aware of therapy myths. For example, knitting does not necessarily increase spasticity.

Finally

Evidence suggests that patients with a stroke spend long periods of time in hospital doing nothing (Lincoln et al, 1989). This time could be used constructively to encourage leisure participation and hence enhance quality of life. Occupational therapists are ideally placed to be involved in such programmes.

Work

The initial period of rehabilitation following a stroke concentrates on enabling the patient to return home to an environment in which he/she can operate as safely and independently as possible. When the patient first goes home an occupational therapist will work with the patient to create a treatment programme that matches their needs and desires. As part of this process, the patient may express a wish to return to work or to seek alternative forms of vocational employment. In order to draw up an appropriate plan with the patient, the occupational therapist should be clear in his/her own mind as to what the term 'work' means.

Standard dictionary definitions are not adequate in describing the role of work as they do not address the complexity of issues surrounding employment. Work is often only associated with paid employment, whereas unpaid work may be of equal importance to the individual. Unpaid work may include such areas as voluntary work or being on a committee. Both paid and unpaid work fulfil a diversity of needs for the individual and some of the many benefits of work are listed below:

- increase in self-esteem;
- maintenance of routines and habits;
- participation in a productive activity;
- involvement in a socially accepted role that provides value to the community;
- having 'a reason to get up in the morning';
- challenging someone to expand their horizons.

By facilitating the patient to take part in a work experience, the occupational therapist acknowledges the above benefits and therefore plays a valuable role in enhancing the well-being of the person.

The occupational therapist can assist the patient in establishing realistic goals and expectations relating to work, and a written joint plan of action should be formulated. As work impinges on others around the individual, family and carers can take an active role in the discussion around work and the plan of action. If returning to a previously held job, the patient will need to break down its components. The joint plan of action can then reflect the skills required to carry out the work. For example, the patient may require further treatment, e.g. improving stamina, in order to be at a level to enter the work environment. Contact with the employer at an early stage is important, in order to establish links and to gain the employer's view, needs and expectations concerning the issue of starting work.

Complications may arise when considering return to work. For example, the employer may not be able to reinstate the person in their workforce. In all cases it is essential to be aware of the issues surrounding the return to work. Liaising with PACT (see below) and other agencies such as unions or occupational health departments may be a prominent feature of the therapist's involvement.

Most occupational therapy departments do not have the specialized equipment required to carry out standardized work assessments, as this is both expensive and space consuming. The Employment Service can carry out work assessments, because they employ a specialist team to work with people with disabilities. Most Job Centres have a Disability Employment Adviser (DEA) forming part of a professional team called PACT (Placing, Assessment and Counselling Team).

PACT provides a service for both those who are returning to work and those who are looking to enter the workforce. As well as providing a work assessment service they can advise on training to update and gain new skills, and work opportunities in a supported environment. If the person is already in employment they will liaise with the employer, assess the work environment and assist with the purchase of necessary, specialized equipment. They will also support the employee back into work. The occupational therapist should contact the local Job Centre for further details.

However, entering the paid work environment may not always be realistic, feasible or desired by the individual. Looking into the voluntary sector may be an alternative solution. In this case contact should be made with a target organization to discuss what positions are available and how appropriate they are to the individual. Again, the components of the tasks to be undertaken need to be analysed and a plan of action made.

How long the occupational therapist lends support to the patient in paid or unpaid employment is at the therapist's discretion. The decision can only be made in the light of detailed knowledge of the patient's individual circumstances. The most important point is to ensure that both the individual and the employer feel confident about the new arrangement. The occupational therapist should therefore provide close support to each party throughout this next phase of the patient's reintegration into the community.

Since 1 October 1999, the Disability Discrimination Act now requires organizations to:

- review their practices, policies and procedures and change any that make it unreasonably difficult for a disabled person to access any of their services;
- review the information given out to patients, visitors and other members of staff, and how staff communicate with patients, visitors and other members of staff, including the provision of auxiliary aids and services;
- review the physical access to all services and, if an area is inaccessible, provide alternative access to services.

Driving

In the UK there is no set procedure for the assessment of drivers who have suffered from a stroke.

- Individuals are not allowed to drive for one month following a stroke, but can return to driving when their clinical recovery is considered satisfactory.
- The person should only return to driving after one month if they are free of any problems that would cause a danger to him/herself or other road users, for example:
  - damage to his/her vision;
  - problems with memory or concentration;
  - slow reactions in an emergency;
  - spasms in a paralysed limb which cannot be controlled;
  - fits or convulsions;
  - certain speech and reading difficulties.

  Advice/guidance *MUST* therefore be sought from the individual's consultant or general practitioner.
- It is the patient's responsibility to advise the DVLA (Driver and Vehicle Licensing Agency, Swansea) but it is usually the GP who decides on fitness to drive.
- GPs receive advice from the DVLA by way of a handbook *Medical Aspects of Fitness to Drive* (Table 5.1). This book gives general advice but no guidance on what to assess; this is left up to the GP's judgement and skill. Comprehensive assessment is rarely carried out. A GP may assess visual and physical impairments within the confines of the surgery but cognitive ability is often overlooked.
- When the DVLA has been notified of the patient's wish to return to driving, it will send a 'medical in-confidence form' to the patient. This will ask for more medical details of the patient's disability and ask for permission for the patient's GP or consultant to make a report to the department's medical advisers. It is a legal requirement for the patient to complete and return this form, otherwise his/her licence may be revoked.
- A medical adviser will consider this report and make a recommendation about the continuation of the patient's licence. The licence will either be granted or revoked. Further assessment from an independent doctor may be requested.
- Research has suggested that cognitive ability plays a vital role in driving performance after brain damage (Nouri et al., 1987). However, there remains conflicting evidence about what cognitive impairment needs to be assessed and what is predictive of driving outcome.
- If there is any doubt about the patient's ability to return to driving, the

following assessments are available:

- cognitive assessment by an occupational therapist or psychologist using the Stroke Drivers Screening Assessment (SDSA) (Nouri and Lincoln, 1994). This is a standardized assessment of the patient's cognitive abilities required for driving. An equation is used which predicts the patient's road test performance. If the patient fails the SDSA, he/she will be advised not to return to driving and to be reassessed approximately 3 months later;
- physical and sometimes cognitive assessment at a mobility centre, which will include assessment for adaptations.

Table 5.1: Medical aspects of fitness to drive (Medical Commission on Accident Prevention)

CVA (cerebrovascular disease, stroke) including stroke due to occlusive vascular disease, spontaneous inter-cerebral haematoma and cerebral ischaemia. TIA (Transient Ischaemic Attack)	*Group 1* At least one month off driving after the event, when clinical recovery and fully satisfactory driving can restart. May be issued with 70 licence provided there is no significant residual disability. If residual limb disability restricted, licence issued endorsed 'with controls to suit disability' (the driver receives separately an explanatory letter 'Driving and Strokes' from the DVLA). Driving should cease until the attack has been controlled for at least three months.

Mobility Centres

Forum of Mobility Centres Accredited Centres

- Banstead Mobility Centre, Damson Way, Fountain Drive, Carshalton, Surrey, SM5 4NR. Tel: 020 8770 1151.
- Cornwall Friends Mobility Centre, Tehidy House, Treliske Hospital, Truro, Cornwall, TR1 3LJ. Tel: 01872 254920.
- Derby Regional Mobility Centre, Kingsway Hospital, Kingsway, Derby, DE22 3LZ. Tel: 01332 371929.
- Disabilities Action, 2 Annadale Avenue, Belfast, BT7 3UR. Tel: 01232 491011.

- Edinburgh Driving Assessment Service, Mobility Centre, Astley Ainslie Hospital, 133 Grange Loan, Edinburgh, EH9 2HL. Tel: 0131 537 9192.
- Kilverstone Mobility Centre, 2 Napier Place, Thetford, Norfolk, IP24 3RL. Tel: 01842 753029.
- Mobility Advice and Vehicle Information Service (MAVIS), 'O' Wing, Macadam Avenue, Old Wokingham Road, Crowthorne, Berks, RG45 6XD. Tel: 01344 661000.
- Mobility Centre, Hunters Moor Regional Rehabilitation Centre, Hunters Road, Newcastle upon Tyne, NE2 4NR. Tel: 0191 219 5694.
- Mobility Information Service, Unit 2A Atcham Estate, Shrewsbury, SY4 4UG. Tel: 01743 761889.
- Wrightington Mobility Centre, Wrightington Hospital, Hall Lane, Wrightington, Wigan, Lancs, WN6 9EP. Tel: 01257 256409.

Associate Members of Forum of Mobility Centres

- The Driving Assessment Service, Hillcrest, Moseley Hall Hospital, Alcester Road, Birmingham, B13 8JL. Tel: 0121 442 3434.
- Irish Wheelchair Association, Blackheath Drive, Clontarf, Dublin 3, Ireland. Tel: 00 3531 8338241.
- Oxford Driving Assessment Centre, Mary Marlborugh Centre, Windmill Road, Headington, Oxford, OX3 7LD. Tel: 01865 227577.

Other Mobility Centres

- Barnsley Regional Mobility Centre, Units 16–18, Mount Osbourne Business Centre, Oakwell Avenue, Barnsley, S71 1HH. Tel: 01226 201101/284710.
- The Donald Tod Rehabilitation Centre, Fazakerley Hospital, Lower Lane, Liverpool, L9 7AL. Tel: 0151 529 3039.
- Disabled Drivers' Voluntary Advisory Service, 18 The Roods, Warton, Lancs, LA5 0QG. Tel: 01524 734195.
- Disabled Living Centre (West of England), The Vassall Centre, Gill Avenue, Fishponds, Bristol, BS16 2QQ. Tel: 0117 9653651.
- Mid Kent Health Care Trust Care Mobility Advice Centre, Preston Hall Hospital, Larkfield Ward, Aylesford, Kent, ME20 7NJ. Tel: 01622 710161 ext. 2241.
- Mid Staffordshire Driving Assessment Service, Cannock Chase Hospital, Brunswick Road, Cannock, WS11 2XY. Tel: 01543 576424.
- North Wales Drivers' Assessments Centre, Ysgol Y Gogarth, Nant Gamar Road, Llandudno, Gwynedd, LL30 1YF. Tel: 01492 872036.
- Rookwood Hospital, Llandaff, Cardiff, CF5 2YN. Tel: 01222 566281.
- Wales Disabled Drivers' Assessment Centre, 18 Plas Newydd, Whitchurch, Cardiff, CF4 1NR. Tel: 01222 615276.

Accidents – Incidence

- Older drivers travel fewer miles than their younger counterparts. Driving experience is more important than age so accident involvement is progressively less with age.
- The highest accident rate per mile is recorded for females aged over 74 years.
- Automatic transmission facilitates adaptation to disabled controls.
- Three-quarters of all strokes occur after 65 years of age.
- Powered steering is an advantage to the older driver as it facilitates parking, though tinted windows should be avoided as they do not reduce glare but visual acuity.
- Joining major roads and turning right are particularly hazardous features for older drivers.
- Taking rear and lateral observations can be difficult as spinal joints may be stiff; American work suggests regular spinal exercises to increase flexibility.
- Giving up driving is not easy for the older driver. Economics show it is cheaper to travel by public transport if annual mileage is below 4000.
- An 18-year-old driver has over three times the accident involvement of the 70-year-old driver.

Sensory Impairment

Normal movement depends on motor and sensory feedback to the brain and central nervous system. This is disrupted following a stroke. Sensory impairment may be evident in the affected side with a lack of feeling in the limb, clumsy movement or poor coordination; for example, inability to pick up keys in pocket without a visual cue.

Cognitive Problems

Concentration/learning/memory

Cognitive problems are evident in many people following a stroke, especially attention and concentration (speed of processing and impaired executive skills) levels, which can have a direct impact on memory and ability to learn new information.

Factors affecting learning ability

- impaired judgement;
- impaired memory;
- reduced imitation;
- reduced concentration (attention);
- impaired reasoning;

- reduced motivation;
- poor task completion;
- perseveration;
- slow speed of processing;
- reduced problem-solving planning;
- impaired higher executive skills (higher level thinking makes new learning more difficult).

Effect of cognitive problems on driving

Often people returning to driving following a stroke may not have driven for a long time before retraining or may be using unfamiliar controls. Therefore it is very probable that they will be anxious during the first few lessons, which will exacerbate or mirror some of these difficulties. Fatigue is another feature following a stroke (mental and physical) that affects the person's ability to learn new skills, especially when facing new situations which demand a lot of physical and emotional energy. Generally people tire as the day progresses.

The road situation is constantly changing, therefore the speed of information processing is highly significant for safe and efficient driving.

Most people can make a correct choice if given unlimited time to observe a situation, but in a moving car, perception of events, decision making and motor actions need to be performed within strict time restraints.

Hints

- Plan lessons for when the person is likely to be performing at his/her best.
- Use structured teaching techniques; for example tasks should be simplified and taught step by step with plenty of opportunity for practice.
- Build up a good relationship with the person. Work on what they know first and build on it.
- Build on positive experience to improve confidence.
- Be consistent with instructions and terms used and make sure the person understands them.
- Use simple instructions and explanations.
- Encourage the individual to keep a diary of his/her achievements and reflect on it (if appropriate, a record of improvements).
- Let the person learn at his/her own rate.
- Provide the individual with feedback on his/her progress and give him/her an understanding of his/her difficulties and capabilities.
- Short, frequent lessons are better than less frequent ones. This minimizes forgetting between lessons and speeds up the learning process.

Visual Perceptual Problems

Research from the Transport and Road Research Laboratory cited human error as the main cause of accidents, specifically those centred around attention, perception and information processing, and visual perceptual errors are the most common.

Visual perception is the process by which the driver makes sense of what he/she does on the road and of the traffic generally. Passive observation of the environment, without recognition of the relevance of what is seen, does not constitute the level of visual attention required for safe driving.

Assuming adequate distance vision, a driver's visual search strategies are the main determinant of what he/she sees and when he/she sees it.

Visual perceptual problems affecting driving

*   inattention: neglect of the affected side of the body or environment;
*   hemianopia: limited visual fields bilaterally;
*   figure–ground problems: difficulty picking out foreground from background;
*   depth and distance problems: difficulty judging depths and distances;
*   spatial orientation difficulties: difficulty judging objects in relation to each other, e.g. road edge to car;
*   right–left discrimination: difficulty distinguishing between left and right.

Visual search, scanning and tracking

Although most visual search is directed at the road ahead, the driver needs to divide his/her attention between the road ahead and events in his peripheral field. Visual search efficiency increases with experience. Often the novice driver spends as much time fixing on the road edge, road markings and objects close to the car as he/she does looking ahead. This is due to uncertainty as to where the most relevant information is likely to be found. This ability to attend to the most informative part of the environment must be learned and will form an important part of the driver's initial tuition.

Hints

These difficulties may lead to positioning problems, i.e. mounting the kerb on the left side without realizing or using white lines in the centre of the road to assist position driving to near centre. If the person has less than 120 degrees of horizontal peripheral vision, he/she should not be driving.

Emotional/Psychological Problems

Often, returning to driving is seen as the key to independence. Owing to the acute nature and trauma of a stroke the residual disabilities can be mild or severe. This does not always proportionally relate to the emotional/psychological impact of the stroke, as everyone is different.

Particular difficulties

- behavioural changes;
- mood;
- personality;
- frustration/anxiety/depression;
- lability;
- relationships;
- financial strain.

Hints

- take a positive supportive approach;
- give encouragement;
- give clear feedback;
- listen.

Communication (Expressive Speech and Understanding)

Communication problems are often involved with damage to the left side of brain and right-sided hemiplegia.

Speech difficulties do not relate to intelligence. Often people know what they want to say but are unable to express themselves. This can lead to frustration for the individual and the instructor.

Hints

- offer reassurance and take time;
- speak clearly, with simple one-part verbal instructions supported by visual cues;
- the individual may be able to write things down;
- he/she may have difficulty in understanding.

Check

- whether the person can follow simple instructions, e.g. check mirror, take off handbrake, turn left;
- whether gestures are needed to clarify verbal instructions;
- whether the person can follow two-part instructions;
- whether the person can understand more complex instructions.

Stroke Education

Stroke is the commonest cause of long-term disability in the western world. Despite this, many patients and their carers are poorly informed about the nature of the illness, recovery, treatment and secondary prevention. Stroke education not only provides information about the illness but empowers individuals by allowing great self-determination, reducing anxiety and improving coping strategies.

Common anxieties include:

- nature of stroke;
- fear of recurrence;
- degree of recovery;
- memory/communication problems;
- driving/fatigue;
- service provision.

Studies (Hanger et al., 1998) have shown that patients continue to ask questions about their condition over prolonged periods of time, i.e. over two years. Wellwood (1994) found large gaps in patients' basic understanding. Occupational therapists often give patients information about stroke but the following need to be considered:

- Is the information given at a time of stress and not retained?
- Is the information fully understood or misinterpreted?
- Cognitive difficulties may lead to impaired retention of information.
- Patients may be unable to take this information on board as they are still adjusting emotionally.

Continuing the education process is essential as the nature of questions changes with time, but the need for information does not.

Chapter 6
Therapeutic Challenges

The Pusher Syndrome and Overuse (Davies, 1985)

Many more patients with left hemiplegia than right suffer from the pusher syndrome. Davies (1985) states that the syndrome in its most severe form is characterized by the following problems:

1. The head is turned to the sound side and is at the same time shifted laterally towards the sound side. When the patient is sitting, he/she is unable to relax his/her muscles in order to allow the head to be side flexed towards the affected side, although it moves freely to the sound side. The eyes are often turned to the sound side as well, and the patient has difficulty in bringing them to the affected side and then maintaining their position.

2. The patient's ability to perceive incoming stimuli from his/her affected side is reduced in all the perceptual modalities, i.e. tactile, visual or auditory.

3. Lying supine on a plinth or in bed, the patient shows an elongation of his/her affected side from head to foot.

4. When lying on the plinth the patient holds onto the edge with his/her sound hand and is anxious that he/she may fall over the side.

5. Placing does not automatically occur when the sound leg is moved, although when asked to hold that leg in a certain position the patient can do so easily.

6. When both knees are flexed with the feet supported on the bed, they lean towards the affected side. A marked resistance is felt when trying to turn both knees to the sound side, i.e. as if to lie them on the bed on that side. No resistance is met when rotating both knees to the affected side.

7. In sitting, the difficulties become more obvious. The head is held stiffly to the sound side and the sound side of the trunk shortens markedly. The affected side is elongated although the weight remains over the

affected side. Resistance is encountered when an attempt is made to transfer the weight over the sound side, with the patient pushing back with the help of his/her sound hand.

8.   Transferring the patient into a chair presents difficulties, as he/she pushes backwards and away from the sound leg.

9.   Sitting in a wheelchair he/she adopts a typical posture. His/her trunk is flexed, his/her head is turned to the sound side and his/her sound arm maintains constant activity, pushing on the arm of the chair.

10. When leaning forwards in order to stand up or transfer into bed, the patient pushes towards the affected side, although his/her trunk is markedly shortened on the sound side. His/her affected foot may slide back under the chair or show no activity at all.

11. In standing, the patient's whole centre of gravity is to the affected side, so that a line drawn from his/her sound foot to his/her sternum would be diagonal to the floor.

12. The patient either leans back against the therapist's supporting arm or flexes his/her trunk forward from the hips and fails to come upright at all.

13. If it is possible to walk with the patient, the affected leg adducts so strongly that it may even cross over in front of the other leg as it is brought forward.

14. As the patient walks towards his/her chair or the plinth, supported by the therapist, he/she sits down prematurely. He/she grasps the arm of the chair and starts sitting down when he/she is still inappropriately far away.

15. Those patients who have no aphasia tend to talk a great deal and offer many explanations for their failure in performance. They require constant verbal instructions from the therapist although the situation would seem to be sufficient.

16. The patient has considerable difficulty in learning to dress him/herself and in activities of daily living in general.

17. His/her sound hand appears clumsy when he/she tries to perform skilled tasks, even though it is often his/her dominant hand.

18. Many perceptual problems are experienced by patients manifesting the pusher syndrome, and will need to be treated accordingly.

Aims of Treatment

1.   Restore movements of the head.
2.   Reduce over-activity (pushing) in sound side.
3.   Assess and treat underlying problems.
4.   Regain the midline in all positions and activities.

Overuse

The pusher syndrome, as described above, is rarely seen in its true form. However, many patients compensate for the lack of function in their affected side by overusing their sound side. This effect mimics the pusher syndrome. Treatment for overuse therefore follows similar lines to that of the pusher syndrome.

Application to Occupational Therapy

1.   Transfer the patient to the sound side to encourage him/her to take his/her weight over to the sound side.

2.   When dressing, have the clothes on his/her sound side. If possible put them on a chair in front and to the sound side, making him/her reach to pick up his/her clothes, therefore taking his/her weight to the sound side.

3.   The patient may be unable to cross his/her affected leg over his/her sound leg to put his/her lower garments on. Therefore teach him/her to cross his/her legs at his/her ankles and reach forwards to put on these garments. This also encourages him/her to lean forwards to the sound side. Alternatively, he/she may have to put his/her sound leg in first to break the pushing.

4.   When standing to pull clothes up, ask the patient to reach his/her sound arm to a point on his/her sound side at shoulder level (this could be to the assistant's hand). This will elongate his/her trunk on the sound side, prevent him/her from leaning backwards and assist in maintaining standing balance.

5.   Encourage the patient to move his/her head to look at an object, to restore movements of the head.

6.   Carry out activities in standing as much as possible to encourage extension in his/her leg and trunk. A plaster of Paris backslab may be needed for the affected leg initially. Encourage the patient to reach up with his/her sound hand, elongating his/her trunk on the sound side, e.g. when combing hair, shaving, taking cups out of a high cupboard to make tea, playing elevated games on the sound side either attached to a wall or on a high table. The therapist should stand on the affected side to ensure that his/her weight is taken over both legs but stimulation, such as verbal instruction, should always come from directly in front of the patient. This needs to be explained to the relatives also.

7.   Climbing stairs with a handrail on the sound side teaches the patient the necessary movements required and usually improves his/her walking immediately afterwards.

8.   Give the patient as much tactile information as possible from the environment, as his/her own feedback system is disturbed. However, bear in mind that if stimulation is given incorrectly, this may increase the pushing, so be careful.

The Shoulder–Hand Syndrome (Davies, 1985)

Davies describes the shoulder–hand syndrome as being a sudden development of a swollen painful hand associated with a subluxed/neglected
shoulder and affects about 12.5% of patients, most commonly between the
first and third month following onset of the stroke. Some 60–80% of patients
suffer from a painful shoulder and the 12.5% who suffer a shoulder–hand
syndrome generally fall within this group. This painful condition interferes
with the patient's overall rehabilitation and if untreated can lead to a permanent fixed deformity of the hand and fingers.

Symptoms

Davies (1985) states that the patient's hand quite suddenly becomes swollen,
and a marked limitation of range of movement occurs rapidly. The oedema is
predominantly apparent on the dorsum of the hand, including the metacar-
pophalangeal joints, and also in the fingers and thumb. The skin loses its
creases, particularly over the knuckles and the proximal and distal interphalangeal joints. The oedema is soft and puffy and usually ends just proximal to
the wrist joint. The tendons of the hand cannot be seen. The colour of the
hand changes, having a pink or lilac hue, which is particularly noticeable if
the arm is left hanging down at the patient's side. The hand feels warm and
sometimes moist. The nails start to undergo changes and appear whiter or
more opaque than those of the other hand.

Loss of passive supination with pain is usually felt at the wrist. Dorsal
extension of the wrist is limited and pain is experienced on the dorsal aspect
when an attempt is made to move passively into an increased range. The pain
is also elicited during weight-bearing activities in therapy, when the arm is
extended and the hand supported flat on the plinth, therefore such activities
should be avoided. There is marked loss of flexion of the metacarpopha-
langeal joints with no bony prominences visible. Abduction of the fingers is
very restricted and the patient has increasing difficulty in clasping his/her
hands together. The fingers of the sound hand appear to be too large to fit
into the spaces between the fingers of the other hand.

The proximal interphalangeal joints are stiff and enlarged. Very little
flexion is possible and there is a loss of full extension as well. Pain is experienced when attempts are made to flex the joints passively. The distal
interphalangeal joints are extended and there is little or no flexion possible.
Even if these joints have stiffened in slight flexion, any attempt at passive
flexion is painful and limited.

Causative Factors

Very little has been convincingly postulated or proved as to the cause of this
syndrome. Something specific must occur that triggers it off and it is then

only perpetuated by the inactivity and the dependent position of the arm. A logical hypothesis is that a mechanical happening causes a primary oedema or an oedema secondary to trauma, and the inadequate muscle pump fails to resolve it. The vicious cycle of oedema, pain, loss of range of movement and sympathetic nervous system involvement follows. Various causes of the oedema in the hand could precipitate the shoulder–hand syndrome:

- prolonged plantar flexion of the wrist under pressure;
- overstretching of the joints of the hand may produce an inflammatory reaction, with oedema and pain;
- fluid from an infusion may escape into the tissues of the hand;
- minor accidents may happen to the hand.

Prevention

Prevention of the shoulder–hand syndrome aims at avoiding all the causes of oedema of the hand.

Treatment

The best results are achieved if the treatment is started in the early stages of the condition, as soon as the oedema, pain or loss of range of movement is observed:

- *positioning*: correct positioning of the shoulder and arm at all times in appropriate alignment, including additional pillows under the arm for added elevation and comfort;
- *avoiding flexion at the wrist*: making a cock-up splint from plaster of Paris, to support the wrist in a comfortable amount of dorsal flexion. The patient should wear this both night and day;
- *compressive centripetal wrapping*: of the digits or extremities has proved to be a simple, safe and dramatically effective treatment for reducing peripheral oedema and its deleterious concomitants. This is used rarely at present but soft tissue massage in elevation is more commonly seen;
- *ice*: immersing the patient's hand in a bucket containing a mixture of ice and water, ideally one-third water and two-thirds ice. Check integrity of sensation prior to this procedure;
- *active movements*: should be performed in therapy whenever possible, rather than passive movements;
- *passive movements*: a careful passive range of movement prevents the shoulder from becoming painful, and passive movements to the hand and fingers should be performed very gently, so as not to produce any pain;
- *oral cortisone*: if the symptoms remain marked and the patient has some activity in the hand, and future function is in jeopardy, oral cortisone can be effective.

Motor Planning and Dyspraxia

Motor Planning

Praxis is the ability to use our limbs and body in skilled tasks in order to function. Practic ability (normal motor planning) involves three stages:

- *ideation*: forming the concept and knowing what to do;
- *motor planning*: organizing the sequence of movement involved in the task;
- *execution*: carrying out the planned movement in a smooth sequence.

To achieve a particular movement a set of motor commands is required. This is called a *motor programme*. The motor programme determines the correct force, direction and timing of the movement. Once motor programmes are learned they become automatic and are laid down as memory traces (motor engrams).

Schmidt (1975) described generalized motor programmes, which are activated for all movements associated with a motor pattern. These are called *movement schemes*, e.g. a motor scheme for reaching and grasping may be used to:

- reach for a cup on the table;
- reach for a tin in the cupboard;
- reach for a child's hand.

The difference of the motor programme is in the force, direction and timing of the movement. More recently Norman (1981) has extended the concept of a single motor programme to an *action schema* which contains all the sensory and motor components of an activity sequence. An action schema develops with practice and experience. An action schema is triggered by input from the environment or from volition. Sequences of subschema are then activated to complete an activity and reach a goal. For example, an action schema for making tea will activate a subschema for fill kettle, switch on, select cup, add tea bag and so on. Attention is demanded to trigger the schema, but the lower level schema proceed automatically unless the environment changes.

Repetition of a motor pattern in all activities that incorporate it, helps the motor scheme become established. This supports the practice of incorporating normal movement patterns into early stages of learning post-injury.

A movement may be initiated by verbal input (commands), visual or tactile input, or by volition. Any action plan involves motor programmes, which are executed in a particular sequence in order to reach a goal or complete a task.

Each action has a sequence, which we may at times perform incorrectly when attempting to achieve a goal, e.g. putting the water in the teapot before putting in the tea, or not putting the car in gear before pressing the accelerator. We have the ability to recognize these errors and compensate for them.

When planning a task, actions are combined with object usage and function. The object and action related to it must match.

Dyspraxia

Dyspraxia comprises disorders of the execution of learned movement, which cannot be accounted for by weakness, incoordination, sensory loss, or by incomprehension of or inattention to commands. Classifications of dyspraxia have been widely discussed in the literature. Liepmann (1905) first described a distinction between ideomotor and ideational dyspraxia.

Other types of dyspraxia have been described, such as dressing dyspraxia and constructional dyspraxia. More recently, however, it has been felt that these are names for the functional outcome of ideational or ideomotor dyspraxia or other performance breakdowns and should not be given individual classifications. We may have an influx of names for any type of task that breaks down in the motor planning stage, for instance, a combing-the-hair dyspraxia or a making-a-cup-of-tea dyspraxia. For these reasons, it is considered that working with these two types of dyspraxia would be of most benefit to occupational therapists.

Ideational Dyspraxia

This is a disorder in the performance of skilled activity because the concept is not understood. It is a disturbance in the conceptual organization of actions. Single actions may at times be performed automatically in a familiar environment. Miller (1986) described several characteristic performance errors, which may be seen in the person with ideational dyspraxia:

- *Elements occur in the wrong order*: The person may pour water into the cup before putting the tea in.
- *Sections of the sequence may be omitted*: The kettle is switched on with no water inside.
- *Two or more elements may be blended together*: The sugar is spooned into the cup whilst also making a stirring motion.
- *The action remains incomplete*: The person may take one cut/slice at a piece of meat and try to eat it even though it has not been completely cut.
- *The action overshoots what is necessary*: The whole cup will be filled with milk instead of a drop sufficient for a cup of tea.
- *Objects are used inappropriately*: A pencil may be used as a comb, or a candle may be struck instead of a match.

- *Movements may be in the wrong plane or wrong direction.*
- *Many of these errors can be interpreted as perseveratory*: After pouring the tea from the pot into the cup, the person may then perform a similar act with the sugar bowl, instead of spooning it in.

Ideomotor Dyspraxia

Ideomotor dyspraxia is a disorder in the initiation and execution of planned sequences of movement. The concept of the task is understood but the movements lack the correct force, direction and timing in order to achieve a motor goal. The person with ideomotor dyspraxia may be able to describe an action and may at times perform it automatically, but will on command be unable to perform a purposeful movement. Miller described performance errors, which are most clearly seen in gestural acts without objects.

These errors relate more to the movement's spatial orientation and trajectory, movement initiation and timing, and distal joint control:

- *Body part as object*: When asked to gesture an action the person may substitute a body part for the object, e.g. using a finger as a toothbrush or a hand as a razor.
- *Altered proximity*: The correct grasp for an action may be displayed, but the movement leaves no space for the pretend implement, e.g. stirring with the hand in the imaginary tea and not above it.
- *Altered plane*: The person may hold the comb flat against the head instead of with the teeth at an angle.
- *Fragmentary responses*: When imitating drinking a cup of tea the person may bring the cup to the mouth but not tilt it.
- *Poor distal differentiation*: There is a failure to produce accurate hand responses even though the arm's overall plane and position are correct.
- *Gestural enhancement*: When gesturing hammering the person may also move his/her head up and down, or rock the body backwards and forwards.
- *Vocal overflow*: Additional noises may accompany an action such as 'bang bang' when gesturing the use of a hammer.
- *Perseveration*: This means that the features of an activity, rather than the whole movement, may be seen in subsequent tasks.

These features may be seen in activities of daily living when the person has difficulty performing motor actions whilst utilizing objects.

Praxis – Motor Planning – Assessment

There is considerable debate in the literature about the assessment of dyspraxia. There are several clinical assessment batteries available but they are generally considered to be non-specific, unreliable and in need of some improvement. At best they can be thought of as crude but useful screening measures (Tate and McDonald, 1995). Many authors have identified verbal command, imitation and object use as the study of a motor plan. There is less work, however, on what constitutes a correct response.

Many studies of ideomotor dyspraxia have used quantitative measurements, for instance scoring on the degree of failure, which provide some information on the severity of the problem, but little on the way in which the performance breaks down. Qualitative measurements of dyspraxia, that is, looking at the type of failure, appear to be more acceptable, for example the analysis of errors.

Occupational therapists can use error analysis in the use of objects as a screening measure for dyspraxia.

Conditions for assessment are verbal command, imitation and object use.

Verbal command

With no object present ask the subject to 'show me how you would':

- wave goodbye;
- brush your teeth;
- erase from a blackboard;
- comb your hair;
- wind up a car window;
- signal 'be quiet'.

Imitation

With the object present, ask the subject to 'show me how you would use this object ... like this, without touching it'. The subject is then presented with a variety of objects, one at a time, which they demonstrate the use of, e.g. hammer, scissors, pen, knife, cup, glass and saw.

Object use

With the object present, ask the subject to 'show me how you would use this object'. The therapist then presents several familiar objects, one at a time, which the subject handles and then performs the action related to the object.

The subject's performance should be observed and errors recorded. The person with ideomotor dyspraxia will perform better when demonstrating with the object in hand and in a familiar environment. The ideational dyspraxic would be poor at imitation, object use and functional use, especially with more than one object. Videoing the patient is often useful to enable an analysis of errors, although consideration should be given as to whether this will exaggerate his/her impairment.

Functional use

The occupational therapist is in the unique position of being able to observe the breakdown of the motor plan in occupational performance, and will be able to determine if, and to what extent, the errors affect the patient's ability.

The assessment of ideational dyspraxia requires the person to perform complex sequential activities. The performance errors should be recorded and compared with the error types described for ideational dyspraxia.

The occupational therapist should observe the subject carrying out a variety of familiar tasks, which include several sequences such as making a hot drink, preparing a snack, or potting a houseplant, to be able to analyse his/her performance. The subject should be familiar with the test environment to ensure this does not influence performance.

As there is little research to say how many error types are needed to conclude the presence of ideomotor or ideational dyspraxia, identification is based on good observation and sound clinical judgement. It is not essential to identify the impairment but it is important to determine how it affects the person's performance.

Many patients are inappropriately diagnosed with dyspraxia when there are underlying physical deficits, in an attempt to explain their poor performance!

Praxis – Motor Planning – Guidelines for Intervention (Jackson, 1999)

General

There is no proven, singular approach to the treatment of dyspraxia. It is a complex problem, each individual having different requirements, and treatment should take this into account.

Some general principles, which can be applied to the treatment of dyspraxia, have been developed from the behavioural learning model which states that treatment should be:

- *Functional*: Treatment should focus on activities that are directly relevant to the patient's lifestyle.
- *Goal based:* Goals are set to maximize the current level of recovery, and should be prioritized according to the patient's and carer's needs.
- *Structured*: This may include breaking down and chaining set routines, which could help ideational dyspraxics to practise a small sequence and gradually incorporate a longer chain of activity.

Treatment should also involve:

- *Errorless Learning*: Learning is more efficient if a trial-and-error approach is not permitted but the person is given cues or prompts, which achieve success and are gradually withdrawn.

- *Generalization*: New skills cannot be expected to generalize, therefore the person must have the opportunity to learn in different relevant environments.
- *Compensation*: Retained capacities should be used to compensate for those lost. It is considered that the use of compensation does not impede the recovery of specific cognitive deficits, including dyspraxia. Research has shown that the impairment itself is not always improved; however, the compensatory strategies taught help the person to function more independently.

Specific procedures

Some specific procedures have been suggested which can be incorporated into an individualized treatment programme:

- *Normal movement*: Facilitation of normal movement patterns by the therapist can help to provide the proprioceptive, tactile and kinaesthetic input during a task, e.g. helping the person's arm through the correct movement to reach for a cup. This is especially appropriate for ideomotor dyspraxics. Once the movement is initiated, the person may be able to go on and complete it.
- *Activities in context*: The patient with ideomotor or ideational dyspraxia is likely to perform better in a familiar environment at an appropriate time of day.
- *Facilitation of automatic activity*: Verbal commands should be kept to a minimum as complex instruction may only serve to inhibit initiation and confuse the person. Indirect commands may help, such as 'Are you thirsty?' rather than 'Pick up the cup'. For ideomotor dyspraxics, the command 'get up' may initiate sit to stand rather than breaking it down into several stages. For ideational dyspraxics, chaining an activity may help to establish its conceptual understanding. If the activity is backwardly chained, the person is facilitated through the activity until the last step and then other steps are gradually introduced.
- *Error recognition*: Some success has been experienced with ideational dyspraxics by teaching them to recognize their own errors and to compensate appropriately. For example, one woman who had ideational dyspraxia repeatedly put her talcum powder in her mouth. Backward chaining was used and she was facilitated through the correct motor plan until her hand was placed on her body to rub the powder in. As more steps were introduced, she was given verbal prompts when an error was made until she was able to carry out the action for herself.
- *Visual imagery*: Ideomotor dyspraxics may find it useful to visually imagine the movement before attempting to carry them out.
- *Support and reassurance*: Patients with ideomotor and ideational

dyspraxia often feel frustrated and stupid. It is important that the therapist explains that they understand they are not being uncooperative and that certain movements are difficult. Achievable activities should always be incorporated into treatment.

Research

Some research currently being carried out in The Netherlands (Van Heugten et al., unpublished) has included the evaluation of a therapy programme for dyspraxia in people who have had a stroke. The assessment and treatment they are evaluating has incorporated the concept of information processing and they describe the performance of an activity as consisting of three stages: initiation, execution and control. The authors felt there was no need for a theoretical distinction between ideational and ideomotor dyspraxia and that it was therefore no longer necessary to distinguish between the two as a starting point for treatment.

Four activities are used for assessment and the observer scores the level of performance. Treatment focuses on performance of activities of daily living and the person is taught to compensate for a dyspraxic movement by altering the way in which the activity is carried out.

Compensation could be internal, for instance, to consciously verbalize the correct stages of an activity, or external, such as choosing alternative fastenings if buttoning a shirt is the problem. As the assessment phase breaks the activity down into three phases of initiation, execution and control, the treatment corresponds to the phase in which the problem occurred.

If initiation is the problem then instruction is given – verbal when minimal problems occur – and if the person is experiencing difficulty initiating the activity, then the therapist may for instance hand objects one at a time to the person. If execution is the problem, specific verbal or physical guidance is given. If the person does not detect or correct performance errors then appropriate feedback is given.

The results of impairment tests indicated small but significant improvements in motor function and dyspraxia. All measurements of disability, however, showed significant improvements in performance of activities of daily living. This indicates that the treatment does not improve the impairment itself but the compensatory strategies taught enable the patient to function more independently. A control group is currently being studied and the final results are being published this year.

Summary

These guidelines recommend the analysis of errors in occupational performance to assess dyspraxia and its effects. Treatment focuses on the subject's ability, by teaching strategies that facilitate more normal motor plans depending on where the performance is breaking down. Dyspraxia remains a controversial and much debated topic and is a challenging area of intervention for occupational therapists. Further research is required to develop assessment tools and treatment strategies, and to investigate their effectiveness.

Dysexecutive Function

Introduction

Luria in 1966 wrote about executive functions, proposing that the frontal lobes were responsible for programming and regulating behaviour.

During the 1980s there was an abundance of literature by many authors, such as Lezak (1982), Kay (1986), Stuss and Benson (1987) and Ylvisaker and Szekeres (1989).

By the 1990s it was clear that deficits in executive functions, more than any other cognitive process, determine the extent of social and vocational recovery.

Sohlberg et al. in 1993 suggested that impairments involving the executive system were often responsible for poor community reintegration.

What are 'Executive' Functions?

The executive system comprises those mental functions necessary for formulating goals, planning how to achieve them and carrying out plans effectively (Lezak, 1982).

It is the process by which we plan, organize, initiate, monitor and adjust our thinking and behaviour (Kay, 1986).

More recently, in 1994, Powell stated that the term 'executive function' described a collection of skills that typify a good administrative executive. The executive is the person who needs to make long-term plans and goals, to organize steps to achieve those plans, to initiate, monitor and subtly adjust those plans when necessary and to have good judgement.

Components of Normal Executive Functioning

The executive system can be broken down and described in several different ways. In 1987, Ylvisaker and Prigatano identified the following items:

- *Realistic goal setting*: This is based on your own awareness of strengths and weakness, knowing what you are capable of achieving. Most humans are goal directed in behaviour.
- *Planning*: Setting out steps to be carried out in a specific order to achieve a task. These steps are related and need to be carried out in a certain order for a successful outcome.

- *Organization*: The way that you carry out the plan. This may involve delegation or acquiring resources.
- *Self-initiation*: The ability to start an activity, for instance a conversation or a task, without a direct command or an external cue. Self-initiation is a spontaneous action.
- *Self-directing*: Once the task is initiated, the ability to carry on with the task without constant feedback and reassurance.
- *Self-inhibiting*: The ability to move or switch attention from one topic to another. This also relates to having appropriate social skills.
- *Self-monitoring/self-correcting*: The ability to monitor if things are going wrong and change them as you go along. Self-correcting is the ability to put something right once it has gone wrong.
- *Flexible problem solving*: The ability to recognize that there is more than one solution to a problem and to think more divergently. Switching attention may well be linked to this area.

Assessment of Executive Functions

Executive functioning is a difficult area to assess. The use of standardized assessments will not always help identify the deficits in this area.

The very act of testing executive control functions may mask an existing impairment. In traditional testing situations the examiner serves, in part, as the patient's executive control system by giving instructions on what to do and when to begin, thereby decreasing and/or eliminating the demands on initiation, planning and organizational processes (Lezak, 1982).

The Hayling and Brixton Test and Behavioural Assessment of Dysexecutive Syndrome (BADS) are examples of standardized assessments. The occupational therapist can undertake a short training course to become a licensed user of these assessments.

Given this complexity of executive functions it is advised that the occupational therapist uses a combination of objective and subjective assessment techniques. It is also of benefit if one can gain access to neuropsychological assessment results. Knowledge of these results will enable discussion of findings to help formulate a hypothesis.

Functional assessment

This is largely clinical observation of skills and behaviours within the patient's prevailing environment. Generally these are not standardized or normalized to populations but tailored to the individual.

Unstructured scenarios such as planning a trip and going on it, and multi-step tasks such as preparing a complicated meal or organizing a cupboard, can be useful in assessing this area. Also it is useful to get the patient to predict how well he/she will complete the task and how long he/she estimates it will take him/her. On completion of the task, give feedback on how long the individual actually took and how well he/she did.

It is vital that tasks are well planned, giving the patient adequate challenge. A routine task such as getting washed and dressed or making a hot drink will not challenge the 'executive system'. The individual needs to utilize prior knowledge but also be exposed to novel situations if possible.

Evaluation of premorbid and current status

It is essential to investigate relevant social, intellectual, emotional and executive function history to establish not only premorbid status but also current status in real-life situations. Interviews with family members can be carried out.

Treatment Approaches in Dysexecutive Function

The literature all suggests that there is no cure for dysexecutive problems and that the use of strategies will perhaps give the best outcome. Two of the more popular approaches used are the folowing.

Prosthetic environments and supports

This approach provides varying amounts of external management and direction. The more severely affected patients may need a tightly controlled environment and continuous supervision to compensate for disorganization.

Often patients will require a prosthetic environment for safety, as well as to enable self- direction and monitoring.

Other supports for less severe problems could be as simple as checklists. These have been very successful in work programmes with work coaches in the USA.

Feedback sheets are also useful for both the therapist and patient to complete and compare. These work on increasing awareness and monitoring actions. In order to use them a degree of mental flexibility is necessary.

Skill-based learning

This is generally the preferred method because it enables the therapist to teach a patient how to deal with problematic situations:

- Teaching the patient how to identify cues of maladaptive behaviour.
- Developing new strategies to compensate for decreased ability (this could involve some of the prosthetic supports discussed above). Work very closely with the patient to facilitate his/her own thoughts on what his/her own behaviour should be in each situation, to avoid the patient 'distancing' him/herself from the strategies.

• Substituting adaptive behaviours for maladaptive behaviours.

Treatment Examples Using the Ylvisaker Breakdown of the Executive System

Realistic goal setting

After completing a task get the patient to write down his/her strengths and weaknesses, and compare these with the therapist's lists. Ask the patient how long the task will take, then compare the length of time it took at the end of the task.

Planning

Give the patient a goal to reach, comprising 7–8 steps. Get him/her to write down how he/she would meet the goal, and have to hand a structured sheet to help with this if necessary.

Organization

Set tasks where the patient needs to carry out the plan, and try to base this on the patient's previous experience. If the patient was used to organizing trips get him/her to plan and organize a trip.

Self-initiation/self-directing

The therapist and patient could keep a feedback sheet of how many prompts the patient requires when carrying out tasks.

Self-inhibition

Social skills groups are one of the best ways of tackling inappropriate social skills (and could involve initiation). For switching attention encourage divergent thinking by getting patients to think of different topics, such as animals for 60 seconds and then colours. Alternatively, the patient could practise alternating between two or more activities, at times designated by the patient in advance.

Self-monitoring/self-correcting

Try to use feedback to improve self-awareness if this is linked to social skills; again a group setting is most useful. Completing a feedback form at the end of each task and talking it through with the therapist may also improve the patient's self-awareness.

Flexible problem solving

Go through different problem scenarios and get the patient to think of more than one way to tackle the problem. You could try to get him/her to think of alternative solutions to solve the problem. Encourage the patient to research the solutions as broadly as possible

Further reading

Duff JD, Campbell JJ. The regional prefrontal syndrome: a theoretical and clinical overview. Journal of Neuropsychiatry 1994; 8(4): 379–87.

Lezak MD. Newer contributions to the neuropsychological assessment of executive functions. Journal of Head Trauma Rehabilitation 1993; March: 24–31.

Muir-Giles G, Clark-Wilson J. Brain Injury Rehabilitation: A Neurofunctional Approach, Therapy in Practice No. 33. London: Chapman & Hall, 1992. [ISBN 156 593 0525]

Sohlberg M, Mateer C. Introduction in Cognitive Rehabilitation Theory and Practice. New York: Guildford Press, 1989: Ch. 10. [ISBN 0898 627 389]

Ataxia (Edwards, 1996)

Three types of ataxia are described:

- *Sensory ataxia*: seen in diabetic or alcoholic neuropathy conditions;
    - disrupts the afferent proprioceptive input to the central nervous system;
    - symptoms include wide-based stamping gait with eyes fixed to the ground for visual feedback.
- *Vestibular ataxia*: seen in peripheral vestibular conditions or central disorders affecting the vestibular nuclei, e.g. medullary strokes;
    - symptoms include disturbances of equilibrium in standing and sitting;
    - may also be accompanied by vertigo, nystagmus or blurred vision.
- *Cerebellar ataxia* : seen in lesions affecting the cerebellum;
    - symptoms include trunkal ataxia and abnormalities of gait and equilibrium;
    - dysarthria and nystagmus may occur;
    - other symptoms include dysmetria, tremor, dyssynergia and visuo motor incoordination, dysdiadochokinesia, posture and gait.

Treatment of ataxia should be a balance between facilitation of impaired control and the recognition and acceptance of necessary compensation which is needed for function. It is recommended that treatment of this nature is discussed with an experienced therapist. Treatment may include:

- *Sensory ataxia*:
    - substitution by the remaining senses.
- *Vestibular ataxia*:
    - vestibular adaptation facilitated by stressing the relevant system;
    - rollator walking frame as a balance aid.
- *Cerebellar ataxia*:
    - use of weights;

- manual guidance/resistance;
- rhythmic stabilizations;
- gymnastic ball;
- re-education of proximal control and performance of goal directed, multi-joint movements;
- stabilization of the trunk and pelvis during functional activities such as eating, to allow greater freedom of the arms.

Speech and Language Deficits

There are three main communication disorders associated with stroke: dysphasia/aphasia, dysarthria and dyspraxia.

Dysphasia

Dysphasia is a disorder of language which can result in difficulty:

- understanding what is said;
- expressing things verbally;
- reading;
- writing.

Dysphasia results from damage to the language centre in the dominant side of the brain – usually in right-handed people this is the left side.

There are many different patterns of dysphasic impairment. Understanding and expression of language are usually both affected, albeit to varying degrees.

The *speech* of a person with dysphasia may show some of the following features:

- maintained ability to use automatic/social speech, i.e. greetings, or counting by rote;
- yes/no responses which are unreliable, either because the question is not understood *or* because one thing is meant/thought but the reverse is said;
- swearing – usually automatic and unintentional;
- one phrase/word/sound produced whenever speech is attempted;
- repeating back what has been said/asked (often without understanding);
- a retained ability to sing (because it is controlled by the opposite side of the brain);
- fluent speech, 'jargon', which is difficult to inhibit (this may comprise a mixture of meaningful and non-meaningful words or may be just a string of sounds);
- grammatical words, such as: the, a, to, etc., are not used;
- word-finding difficulties – some dysphasics may be able to describe something about a word, but not retrieve the word itself.

The Stroke Association publishes leaflets with advice helpful to patients and to therapists on how to deal with dysphasia. The occupational therapist should liaise with the speech and language therapist on ways to encourage return of speech whilst carrying out occupational therapy activity with the dysphasic patient, as intensive practice is beneficial. The obvious strategies of writing or signboards should be tried, but are not always helpful. It is vital to the patient that everyone perseveres in trying to understand what he or she is saying. Gestures and cues should be used to assist the patient who has receptive difficulties to enable him/her to participate in treatment. The family or carers should have the situation explained and be involved in developing ways of communicating.

Understanding

Problems understanding language will range in severity from virtually no understanding of spoken language to mild difficulty apparent only when following group conversation or conversation against a noisy background.

When people with dysphasia are having severe difficulties understanding what is said they compensate by looking out for:

- Visual or non-verbal cues:
    - the gestures we use alongside our speech;
    - body language;
    - facial expressions;
    - tone of voice.
- Situational cues:
    - things in the environment which help determine what is being asked, e.g. the tea trolley, drugs trolley etc.

Understanding can be helped by using demonstration and gesture alongside or instead of spoken instructions.

Dysarthria

Dysarthria is a *speech disorder* caused by damage to the nerves supplying the muscles used when speaking. It may involve problems with breath control for speech, voice production, controlling whether air is directed orally or nasally during speech, and articulation of speech sounds.
It can range in severity from mildly slurred speech to inability to produce any intelligible speech.
Because his/her language skills are intact, a person with dysarthria is often able to use *alternative means of communication*, for example:

- writing;
- spelling words out on an alphabet chart;
- using an electronic communication aid.

Verbal Dyspraxia

This is a disorder affecting the *purposeful* coordination of muscle movements for speech production. It is not a language problem, but very often people with verbal dyspraxia also have some degree of dysphasia. It is characterized by the following:

- groping/struggling to achieve the correct sounds for a word or to sequence the sounds in the right order;
- awareness of errors and subsequent frustration and repeated attempts;
- speech produced 'subconsciously' or automatically will be noticeably more fluent than purposeful speech;
- the speech muscles are *not* paralysed and automatic movements are retained, e.g. for eating, drinking, laughing.

Communicating with a Dysphasic Person

1. *Face the person* you are talking to and direct your speech to him/her all the time.
2. *Keep the background noise to a minimum*, i.e. turn down the television or radio or take the person to a quieter room.
3. *Alert the person* to the fact that you are talking to him/her. Give him/her time to tune in to listening to you, e.g. use his/her name to focus his/her attention, or touch him/her and pause before speaking, or use a lead-in phrase such as 'I wanted to tell you...'.
4. *Slow down* your rate of speech slightly, but do not over-exaggerate your articulation or shout.
5. *Give time to understand* by presenting information in chunks, one piece at a time, e.g. 'I'll put your glasses ... on the table ... by your bed' and pausing frequently.
6. *Repeat or rephrase* what you have said if you are not understood. Try putting the most important word at the end of the sentence, e.g. 'What is your *address*?'.
7. *Stress or emphasize important words* in the sentence, e.g. 'Did *Christine* ring?' or 'Did Christine *ring*?'.
8. *Give clues about what you are saying*, e.g. use a gesture, or write down important words, or draw attention to a photograph or an object relating to what you are saying.
9. *Do not change topics quickly* – leave plenty of time before moving on to something new and give time to let the dysphasic person tune into the new topic.
10. *Be specific*, e.g. 'I'll put your clothes in the wardrobe', not 'I'll put them there'.

11. *Take time to be a good listener* – keep calm, be alert to the dysphasic person's use of gesture, his/her facial expressions etc., listen and watch out for the intention behind what he/she is communicating, even if the individual words do not make sense.

12. *Encourage methods other than speech* – using gesture, drawing on paper or in the air, writing down the whole or part of a word, pointing to pictures or a choice of written words.

13. *Accept a message conveyed by whatever means is possible* – do not then force him/her to use a 'better' method, e.g. do not ask him/her to repeat 'I want a drink' when he/she has gestured his/her need.

14. *Ask questions to guide you to the general topic*, e.g. 'Is it to do with home?' and use your knowledge of the person's activities, needs and situation to help you guess the topic of conversation.

15. *Let the person know what you have understood.* Summarize what you feel has been said to check you have got it right, e.g. 'I think you are telling me something about dinner'.

16. *Don't pretend to understand.* Ask for more information or repetition if you have not understood. The dysphasic person will soon realize if you are pretending to understand and this is likely to lead to more frustration.

17. *Help the person find a particular word by encouraging him/her to describe something about the word*, e.g. what you do with it, what it looks like etc., or think of something associated with the word, e.g. a word similar in meaning or the category (animal, flower etc.).

Dysphagia

Dysphagia is difficulty in safely moving a bolus of food, or liquid, from the mouth to the stomach without aspirating, and involves the chewing and tongue movement preparing food for swallowing as well as the actual swallow. Apparently, thorough clinical examination will identify dysphagia, but can fail to identify 40–58% of patients aspirating. All staff working with the stroke patient should be aware of the possibility of dysphagia and take appropriate action if they feel someone may be aspirating. Initial severity does not mean that the patient will not recover and reported recovery rates within the first few weeks vary from 43% to 86%.

Signs which may indicate a swallowing problem are:

- loss of food or liquid from the mouth, or drooling;
- difficulty in swallowing saliva, so that drooling is a continual problem;
- food remaining inside the mouth after eating, often pocketed inside a cheek or across the roof of the mouth;
- coughing or choking while eating or drinking;

- change in voice quality after eating or drinking – often the voice sounds wet or gurgly;
- breathlessness after eating or drinking;
- mealtimes taking longer to finish – often there may be weight loss;
- someone may complain of food feeling stuck in the throat;
- frequent pneumonias.

Below is advice for someone with swallowing problems:

- Always sit as upright as possible when eating or drinking.
- Remain upright for 15–20 minutes afterwards.
- Avoid noise or other distractions. Do not try to talk and eat at the same time.
- Sipping iced water or ice cream, or sucking on iced pops before starting a meal may be helpful in stimulating the swallowing mechanism.
- Take smaller mouthfuls of liquids and food. All food should be chewed well.
- Ensure a strong swallow between each mouthful; when possible try a second swallow, or cough to clear the throat.
- Following a stroke someone may tire easily and this may affect the swallow. If mealtimes are taking longer and are tiring, try smaller meals, taken more frequently or with snacks in between.
- If there is a tendency for food to remain in the mouth after eating, clean the mouth after mealtimes with a soft toothbrush or mouthwash.

People with severe dysphagia will be fed through a nasogastric or Percutaneous Endoscopic Gastrostomy (PEG) tube. However, oral feeding is always seen as preferable when possible, and food consistency can be varied to suit the patient's swallowing ability, under the guidance of the speech and language therapist. The patient must be reassessed at regular intervals.

Food and taste play an important part in our lives and the occupational therapist can liaise with the speech and language therapist to work on swallowing with changing tastes and food consistencies. The therapist should ensure the patient is well seated and supported at mealtimes, encouraging the individual to feed him/herself, and trying to balance dignity with cleanliness! The Stroke Association leaflet on swallowing difficulties gives good advice on eating.

The therapist should be aware of swallowing difficulties when working on aspects such as cleaning teeth, and making drinks and meals.

It is important that all members of the team stress to the patient the importance of his/her adapted diet to encourage patient acceptance of what often appears unappealing. This is especially true for the patient who has to maintain a special diet after discharge.

Chapter 7
Evaluation

Occupational Therapy Stroke Standards

Standards for stroke care have recently been produced by the Royal College of Physicians and new documentation is also being produced by the College of Occupational Therapy. An example of occupational therapy stroke standards, developed in Nottingham in February 1999, is included below.

Occupational Therapy Standards for Stroke Care in Nottingham Health District

Document prepared by Nottingham Occupational Therapy Stroke Clinical Forum (Judi Edmans, City Hospital, Katharine Hartle and Jenny Bishop, University Hospital, Julie Napper, Highbury Hospital, Jane Balmbra, Lings Bar House and Rachel Keay, Community Rehabilitation), in consultation with all Occupational Therapists in Nottingham treating patients suffering from stroke. Document based on draft occupational therapy standards for stroke care from the Royal College of Physicians.

(A) Role of the Occupational Therapist in Stroke Care

Occupational therapy aims to:

- improve the quality of life of people following stroke at any age, by helping with the practical management of daily life;
- promote enhanced occupational performance in the activities of self-care (feeding, dressing, toileting), productivity (homemaking, employment) and leisure (voluntary work, hobbies, sports).

The occupational therapist will:

* assess the person's level of residual or potential skill;
* analyse the pattern of activities the person needs, wants or is able to do;
* help the person to establish programmes for managing daily life;
* seek to work with the person to support him/her in achieving his/her goals in his/her chosen environment, which may be the home, the workplace, the family or the wider society.

The basic criterion for treatment by an occupational therapist is not the level of impairment caused by a stroke, but rather the level of disability and handicap displayed by a person in daily life activities, i.e. self-care, productivity or leisure. An occupational therapist will need to treat a person where there is only a mild level of physical impairment but where there are marked cognitive, perceptual or emotional problems affecting function.

Occupational therapy practice crosses the geographical boundaries of primary and secondary health care. The occupational therapist will assess the patient's environment, which may require home or workplace visits and may require continuing rehabilitation or review after discharge into the community.

It is not acceptable practice for occupational therapists to be used solely to provide equipment to speed discharge from hospital.

Patients requiring outpatient occupational therapy should be offered the choice of treatment in outpatient occupational therapy departments in hospital, day hospital or in the community. Existing services do not show evidence of equity of care across Nottingham but all three types of outpatient follow up should be available to all patients within the Nottingham Health District.

At present there is a paucity of occupational therapy research to guide evidence-based practice. There are few accredited training courses in neurology for occupational therapists to demonstrate and share higher levels of experience and skill.

(B) Standards of Practice in Occupational Therapy

All occupational therapists are expected to know and work to the following documents. This will result in occupational therapists working to a high standard of practice.

College of Occupational Therapists code of ethics and professional conduct:

* Patient autonomy and welfare
* Personal/professional integrity

- Professional competence and standards
- Service to patients

College of Occupational Therapists standards, guidelines, policies, procedures documents:

- Audit
- Consent for occupational therapy
- Data Protection Act
- Guidelines for documentation
- Home visiting with hospital inpatients
- Individual performance review
- Induction
- Manual handling operations regulations 1992 and their application within occupational therapy:
- Occupational therapy in private practice
- Occupational therapy services for consumers with physical disabilities
- Professional negligence and litigation
- Setting up a quality-assurance programme
- Statement on occupational therapy referral
- Statement on supervision in occupational therapy
- Therapeutic intervention by occupational therapists with consumers in their own homes

(C) Specific OT Standards for Stroke Care in Nottingham

The Nottingham Occupational Therapy Stroke Clinical Forum has written these standards based on their expert opinion of good practice. The group acknowledges that not all of these standards are achievable within the current resources in Nottingham.

1. Organization

Standard 1.1

There will be an occupational therapy service agreement for stroke patients within each trust, which details: access, staffing and location of service provision and nature of the occupational therapy service.

Standard 1.2

The occupational therapy stroke service within each trust will be under the overall supervision of a senior occupational therapist with at least five years' experience, of which at least three will be in neurology.

Standard 1.3

All occupational therapists in stroke care will receive supervision at regular intervals by a senior occupational therapist experienced in neurology.

Standard 1.4

It is expected that an occupational therapist working in stroke care will be a member of the relevant College of Occupational Therapists specialist section, i.e. National Association of Neurological Occupational Therapists (NANOT) or Occupational Therapy for Elderly People (OCTEP), to ensure access to updated knowledge, courses and peer networking.

Standard 1.5

There will be written evidence of formal links and communication by the occupational therapy service with other statutory and voluntary services specifically relating to stroke patients' continuing care (e.g. local authority, Stroke Association).

2. Patient Care

Standard 2.1

Following referral, initial assessment will be commenced within an agreed time-scale:

Inpatients in hospital	1 working day
Outpatients in hospital	1 week
Outpatients in day hospital	1 week
Community rehabilitation	1 week

All patients who have suffered a stroke should be referred for occupational therapy. General practitioners and hospital consultants must be aware that the referral has been made.

Standard 2.2

All patients will have a named occupational therapist.

Standard 2.3

Written information on occupational therapy will be given to the patient and family, including details of their named occupational therapist.

Standard 2.4

Consent will be gained from the patient or carer for occupational therapy assessment and intervention.

Standard 2.5

All patients referred will be assessed for occupational therapy intervention. Former and present function will be assessed in terms of self-care, productivity and leisure, for example:

- activities of daily living
- perceptual and cognitive abilities
- home circumstances
- mobility (transfers and wheelchair)
- driving
- employment
- leisure
- splinting

Standard 2.6

Standardized assessments will be used to assess perceptual and cognitive abilities. These may include Rey Figure copying assessment, Rivermead Perceptual Assessment Battery, Middlesex Elderly Assessment of Mental State, Stroke Drivers Screening Assessment.

Standard 2.7

A goal-orientated treatment plan will be developed following the assessment, in negotiation with the patient or carer. Occupational therapy or multidisciplinary goals will be written down, with a copy given to the patient.

Standard 2.8

The treatment plan will be discussed by the multidisciplinary team, patient and carer with target dates, e.g. at case conferences or in medical notes:

Inpatients in hospital	Weekly
Outpatients in hospital	Fortnightly
Outpatients in day hospital	Monthly
Community rehabilitation	Monthly

Standard 2.9

If a treatment need is identified, the treatment will be available:

Inpatients in hospital	Five days per week
Outpatients in hospital	Five days per week
Outpatients in day hospital	Each attendance
Community rehabilitation	Three days per week

Standard 2.10

Treatment will be offered in the areas of: activities of daily living, perceptual and cognitive abilities, mobility, return of upper limb function, splinting, work, leisure, driving, home visits, group work or sensory retraining.

Standard 2.11

Carers will be given the opportunity to participate in the patient's treatment with the patient's consent and this will be documented.

Standard 2.12

Carers will be taught any appropriate techniques required for the care of the patient and this will be documented.

Standard 2.13

Education, support and advice will be provided to carers and this will be documented.

Standard 2.14

The goal-orientated treatment plan will be reviewed and evaluated regularly, involving discussion with the patient and carer, with a written copy given to the patient or carer. This will either be occupational therapy only or, whenever possible, will be multidisciplinary.

Inpatients in hospital	Weekly
Outpatients in hospital	Monthly
Outpatients in day hospital	Monthly
Community rehabilitation	Six-weekly

Standard 2.15

Discharge will be planned with the multidisciplinary team involving the patient and carer, and this will be documented.

Standard 2.16

A written discharge summary/report will be completed. This will include an outline of the patient's functional level, equipment required and supplied, home visit report and plans for future treatment.

Standard 2.17

The patient will be given a copy of his/her own discharge plan.

Standard 2.18

The patient will be given written information on how to contact occupational therapy for information in the future.

Standard 2.19

The patient will be given information on accessing community resources.

3. Documentation

Standard 3.1

Accurate documentation will be written on each patient's occupational therapy assessment and intervention.

Standard 3.2

Patients will have a copy of their rehabilitation goals.

Standard 3.3

Patients will have a copy of their follow-up plan.

4. Training

Standard 4.1

All occupational therapists involved in stroke care will be taught appropriate manual handling skills, by an occupational therapist experienced in neurological occupational therapy, before manually handling a patient. This will follow the College of Occupational Therapists guidelines on manual handling operations regulations 1992 and their application within occupational therapy.

Standard 4.2

All occupational therapists involved in the assessment and treatment of patients following stroke will have access to and be committed to ongoing continuing professional development in neurological occupational therapy.

Methods of Recording Occupational Therapy Intervention

Occupational Therapy case notes can take many forms across a variety of clinical settings. They can either be unidisciplinary or multidisciplinary. Three of the most commonly used are problem-orientated medical records, goal-directed notes and integrated-care pathways.

Problem-Orientated Medical Records (POMR)

These were developed by Dr Lawrence Weed, University of Vermont, USA, in 1969. The notes consist of four sections: database, problem list, progress notes (SOAP – subjective, objective, analysis, plan) and discharge summary. The database contains personal and medical information about the patient. The problem list numbers the specific problems to be addressed by the occupational therapist. The progress notes are only recorded when there is a change or there is some relevant information to be added. Progress is recorded under four headings: *subjective* includes information obtained from the patient; *objective* is the therapist's clinical observations and results of assessments/measures; *analysis is* the therapist's professional opinion of what happened during a treatment session; finally, *the plan* is what will be done next. The discharge summary is placed in the final progress notes and should contain information on personal/domestic activities of daily living, mobility, transfers, cognition, perception, communication, upper limb function, current problems and future care.

Goal-Directed Patient Records (GDPR)

There are many types of goal-directed notes used by occupational therapists on a unidisciplinary and multidisciplinary basis. Goal setting is now commonly used in stroke rehabilitation within the multidisciplinary team. Goal planning should actively involve the patient and family/carers. Once the multidisciplinary team has completed its specific assessments, the patient's problems and needs can be identified, focusing on his/her strengths rather than his/her weaknesses. Long-term and short-term goals can be set. A goal must be related to a change in behaviour, be patient-centred, and be specific, measurable, achievable, realistic and timely (SMART). When writing a goal, it should clearly state who the subject is, what he/she will do, under what conditions, in what time period and what defines a successful outcome. The outcome of a goal can be scored in three possible ways: achieved, partially achieved or not achieved. If the outcome is one of the latter two, then a variance code can be applied to explain the reasons why this is the case. These codes can include issues relating to the patient, care or staff and internal or external factors.

   Another method of goal setting was described by Cook and Spreadbury in 1995 in 'Measuring the outcomes of individualized care'. Goal-directed patient records have been adapted from POMR. Goals are chosen by the patient instead of listing problems, and are agreed in a contract between him/herself and the occupational therapist. However, the therapist may need to write the goals if the patient is unrealistic or has communication problems. ACTOR (activity, patient's observations, therapist's observations, overall evaluation, replanning) headings are used for the progress notes.

Activity includes the facts of the activity; patient's observations are his/her subjective comments; therapist's observations are objective comments on the therapy carried out; overall evaluation is the analysis of treatment; finally, replanning is the future plan which has been set as a result of the treatment session.

Integrated Care Pathways

Integrated care pathways are a well-established method of recording care on a multidisciplinary basis, with patients, following hip replacement or fractured neck of femur. They have also been used in the care of patients following myocardial infarction and a variety of surgical and gynaecological procedures. This form of documentation is now being used by multidisciplinary teams treating patients following stroke.

An integrated care pathway is a record of care that focuses on agreed intervention and expected outcomes for a given patient diagnosis, symptom or procedure, within an identified time frame. It should be developed and written by the multidisciplinary team involved with the delivery of care to the patient. All professionals involved should have common understandings and ownership of the pathway. Outcomes must be agreed, achievable and evaluated at every stage. The documentation replaces all existing notes used by each profession. An integrated care pathway focuses on the 'routine' rather than the exception. When a detour from the care pathway occurs, a variance code is recorded. The four codes relate to the patient's condition, the patient/family circumstances, the clinical and the internal/external systems.

In order for the implementation of an integrated care pathway to be successful, a total review of care delivery is required: organizational, training, development, effectiveness, quality, information and communication.

Integrated care pathways can facilitate best practice and aid multidisciplinary communication. They can also be used for research, clinical audit and as a risk-management tool.

An example of an integrated care pathway for stroke rehabilitation on the Nottingham Stroke Unit has previously been published (Edmans et al., 1997).

Pros and Cons of Multidisciplinary Joint Documentation

Positive reasons for joint documentation:

- to reduce duplication of notes, e.g. front sheets/database, medical history, social history, case conference information, family case conference information, discharge plans, washing and dressing, bathing, transfers, walking, home visits etc., as only one set of notes is written;
- to have easier access to each other's notes, as there is only one set and therefore it is in one place, i.e. all information about the patient is centralized;

- to improve communication, as information written in one place by all of the multidisciplinary team;
- to have one comprehensive set of notes;
- to reduce case conference note taking as only one person needs to write them, giving more opportunity for the lead of the case conference to be rotated around all disciplines;
- to improve goal setting as goals set weekly at case conference;
- to be better for patients as there will be more time for treatment and less repetition of staff asking patients for the same information;
- to have more focused care planning;
- to improve handover of information between disciplines;
- to have a more coordinated discharge;
- to follow on from care pathways;
- *OVERALL EACH PERSON SHOULD WRITE LESS NOT MORE.*

Negative reasons for joint documentation:

- difficulty keeping notes up to date currently but will ensure everyone keeps up to date;
- where to keep notes – currently separate notes:
  - nurses – by bedside and at nurses' station;
  - OT, PT, SALT, psychologist – in own treatment rooms and locked up at night;
  - medical – in notes trolley at nurses' station;
- Future joint notes – in medical notes trolley at nurses' station.
- sending information to different departments for outpatient treatment – send copy of discharge summary only;
- staff wanting to write in notes at the same time;
- where to file the notes ultimately – all notes will be filed with main medical notes in medical records;
- differences in style of writing – all staff write in their normal fashion then iron out any problems later;
- will it become a very bulky set of notes – old medical notes to be filed in filing cabinet for reference only until discharge then add joint documentation notes to them;
- will detail be lost in notes – it is up to each discipline to write appropriate details in the notes as normal;
- confidentiality – notes cannot be left at the end of the bed;
- how will different professional heads of department respond;
- how to find notes by own profession if cover being given from another unit/ward etc.

Evidence-based Practice

Definitions

Evidence-based practice

Evidence-based practice is the explicit use of the best evidence of clinical and cost-effectiveness when working with a particular patient. It combines clinical reasoning, existing research evidence and patient choice.

Research

Research is a systematic investigation to increase knowledge about the most effective form of treatment which can be generalized and applied to other populations.

Audit

Audit is a quality process which compares actual performance in a specific setting against agreed standards of practice. Clinical guidelines may be evidence or knowledge based.

Why do we Need Evidence-based Practice?

Evidence-based practice is needed:

- to secure the greatest health gain from the available resources;
- to ensure decisions about clinical services are driven by evidence of efficacy and cost effectiveness;
- to review and monitor interventions with systematic assessment of health outcome.

Action Needed

- Clinicians, managers, patients and educators must be able to access sufficient information to inform their practice.
- It is necessary to transform information into change of practice.
- The NHS should monitor change.

Definitions of Key Concepts

Efficacy: does treatment X do better than treatment Y under ideal controlled conditions?
Effectiveness: does treatment X do better than treatment Y in standard routine practice?
Appropriateness: is this treatment or care worth doing?

Outcome: the end-point of a process which was brought about can be attributed to the prior treatment or care process leading to individual health gain.

Impact: the effect (outcome) of an intervention on the population leading to population health gain.

Delays in Getting Research Findings into Practice

Some examples are:

- lemon juice to prevent scurvy – 300 years;
- thrombolytic treatment for myocardial infarction – 10 years;
- dilation and curettage (D&C) – dismissed as 'therapeutically useless and diagnostically inaccurate' in 1993, but in 1993–94 was still the fourth most common surgical procedure in the NHS.

Stages of Evidence-based Practice

These are:

- primary research into clinical and cost effectiveness of healthcare interventions;
- review and dissemination of research findings;
- application of research findings to influence clinical practice.

Criticisms of Evidence-based Practice

Criticisms relate to:

- finding the evidence;
- quality of the evidence;
- usability of the evidence;
- expertise, i.e. do purchasers have the skills to judge evidence and its clinical application;
- relevance of the evidence, i.e. if it works in 95% of cases, what if your patient is in the other 5%?

Finding the Evidence

This is not without problems:

- Many rehabilitation journals are not included in Medline and accessing AMED is expensive.
- Most rehabilitation journals are not held in medical libraries.

Sources of Evidence

Technical publications

A list of these is given below:

British Journal of Occupational Therapy
American Journal of Occupational Therapy
Canadian Journal of Occupational Therapy
Scandinavian Journal of Occupational Therapy
Journal of Occupational Therapy Practice
Physiotherapy
Physical Therapy Reviews
Clinical Rehabilitation
Disability and Rehabilitation
British Journal of Therapy and Rehabilitation
Evidence Based Nursing

Health service publications

These include:

Effective Health Care Bulletin
Outcomes Briefing Newsletter
Clinical Standards Advisory Group Reports
Bandolier
Health Care Needs Assessment

Organizations

These include:

NHS Centre for Reviews and Dissemination
Cochrane Collaboration
Centre for Evidence Based Medicine
Royal Colleges and COT/CSP
Central Health Outcomes Unit
UK Clearing House for Information on the Assessment of Health Outcomes

Where to Find the Evidence

Sources are:

- the Internet;
- university libraries:
    - Medline;
    - Cinahl;
    - Embase;
    - electronic/hand search;
    - literature searches;
- College of Occupational Therapy;

- clinical audit departments;
- *Bandolier* journal;
- medical/therapy journals;
- books;
- abstracts/proceedings of conferences;
- special-interest groups;
- specialists;
- research institutes – e.g. Trent.

Levels of Reading

These can be classified as follows:

- browsing;
- reading for information;
- reading for research.

Research Articles

These have four main sections (IMRAD structure):

- introduction;
- method;
- results;
- discussion.

Also useful is *A Pocket Guide to Critical Appraisal* by Iain Crombie. London: BMJ Publishing Group, 1998. [ISBN 0 7279 1099 X]

Levels of Evidence

These may be classified as follows:

(1) meta-analysis (statistical summary of effects);
(2) systematic review (following standardized protocols);
(3) randomized controlled trial (RCT);
(4) other intervention trials;
(5) consensus view (expert committees etc.);
(6) clinical experience.

Questions to Ask when Reading a Paper (Crombie, 1998)

Consider the following:
- Is it of interest?
  - title, abstract.
- Why was it done?
  - introduction;
  - background to study;

- reviews of previous work;
- highlight gaps in knowledge;
- state purpose of study/hypothesis.
- Has it been done before?
  - introduction.
- How was it done?
  - method;
  - what data were collected;
  - how data were collected;
  - statistical methods used.
- What has it found?
  - results;
  - tables/figures with text.
- What are the implications?
  - discussion.

Crombie's General Critical Appraisal Questions

- Are the aims clearly stated?
- Was the sample size justified?
- Are the measurements likely to be valid and reliable?
- Are the statistical methods described?
- Did untoward events occur during the study?
- Were the basic data adequately described?
- Did the numbers add up?
- Was the statistical significance assessed?
- What do the main findings mean?
- How are the null findings interpreted?
- Are important effects overlooked?
- How do the results compare with previous reports?
- What implications does the study have for your practice?

Crombie's Specific Checklists

For appraising:

- surveys;
- cohort studies;
- clinical trials;
- case-controlled studies;
- review papers.

Crombie's Checklist for Appraising Clinical Trials

The essential questions

1. Were treatments randomly allocated?
2. Were all the patients accounted for?
3. Were outcomes assessed blind?

The detailed questions

Design

1. Are the aims clearly stated?
2. Was the sample size justified?
3. Are the measurements likely to be valid and reliable?
4. Could the choice of subjects influence the size of treatment effect?
5. Were there ambiguities in the description of the treatment and its administration?
6. Are the statistical methods described?
7. Could lack of blinding introduce bias?
8. Are the outcomes clinically relevant?

Conduct

1. How was randomization carried out?
2. Did untoward events occur during the study?

Analysis

1. Were the treatment groups comparable at baseline?
2. Were results analysed by intention to treat?
3. Was the statistical significance discussed?
4. Were the basic data adequately described?
5. Did the numbers add up?
6. Were side-effects reported?

Interpretation

1. What do the main findings mean?
2. How are the null findings interpreted?
3. Are important effects overlooked?
4. How do the results compare with previous reports?
5. What implications does the study have for your patients?

Reasons why Papers are Rejected for Publication

The main reasons are:

- the authors did not investigate an important scientific question;
- the study had been done before;
- the study did not test the author's hypothesis;
- the wrong methodology was used;
- the sample size was too small;
- the study was uncontrolled;
- the statistical analysis was incorrect;
- the authors made unjustified conclusions;
- the paper was so badly written that it was incomprehensible.

Outcome Measures

There are two main types of outcome measurements, standardized and individualized. Examples of standardized measures are the SF36 (Garret et al., 1993) (which is a health profile), and the Barthel Index (Wade, 1992). These measures have been tested for validity and reliability, over large populations and the scores are published, allowing therapists to compare results with each other. They also allow patients' scores to be compared with a normal range and with other patients who have similar conditions.

Examples of individualized outcome measurement tools include:

- Treatment Evaluation by A. le Roux's Method (TELER) (le Roux, 1993);
- Goal Attainment Scaling (Ottenbacher and Cusick 1990);
- Canadian Occupational Performance Measure (COPM) (Law et al., 1991);
- Patient Orientated Evaluation Method (POEM) (Bassetlaw Physiotherapy Research Group, 1992).

All of these are scaled. Individualized measures are more sensitive to small changes, which may be important to the patient. These measures can be used for all patient groups and allow for very specific outcomes to be measured. Simpler measures include the Binary Individualised Outcome Measure (Cook and Spreadbury, 1995); here the expected outcome has either been achieved or not.

What may Need to be Measured during the Therapy Process?

This usually consists of one or a combination of the following:

- physical/mental health;
- motivation and mood;
- self-esteem;
- skills and coping strategies;
- functional performance (motor, sensory, cognitive, perceptual);
- relationships and roles;
- work and leisure activities;
- activities of daily living.

What are the Directions of Change to be Measured?

These are:

- improvement;
- maintenance, e.g. of function;
- reduction, e.g. of pain or discomfort;
- prevention, e.g. of disability or discomfort;
- development/maturation;
- recovery, e.g. of function;
- delay, e.g. in rate of deterioration.

Outcomes should be:

- comprehensive;
- sensitive to patient's needs and priorities;
- realistically achievable;
- attributable to the therapy being given.

The measurement of outcomes should be able to:

- measure levels of achievement;
- record change over specific time periods;
- measure feelings and attitudes;
- be reliable;
- be valid (does it measure what it says it is measuring, and is it a meaningful outcome for the patient?).

In clinical settings an outcome measure should:

- enhance existing documentation and communication;
- enhance clinical reasoning and decision making;
- be adopted within available resources;
- motivate staff to use the system.

When using individualized outcome measures the following stages should be used:

1. Individualized problems or goals are identified and negotiated with the patient. These indicate the expected outcomes of therapy.
2. A programme of therapy is planned and implemented.
3. Following an agreed time limit of therapy or number of sessions, the actual outcomes are compared with the expected outcome to measure whether therapy has been effective.

As each patient's goals are different it is difficult to ensure that achievement is being measured the same way across many patients. In order to work towards more reliable measurement, it is helpful for peer groups of staff to discuss individual cases and question each other about how they are setting expected outcomes and measuring actual outcomes.

Therapists need to identify those expected outcomes that were planned to be achieved through the therapy process, within the time limit set. The more closely the therapy programme relates to the expected outcome, the more likely is it that the actual outcomes are attributable to the therapy.

Copies of the SF 36 are available from the UK Clearing House for information on the assessment of Health Outcomes, 1993 Outcomes Briefing: The Nuffield Institute for Health, 71–75 Clarendon Rd, Leeds LS2 9PL, UK.

Chapter 8
New Approaches

Restoring Motor Function in the Stroke Upper Limb using Bilateral Isokinematic Training and Electromyographical Biofeedback

Restoration of normal function to the hemiplegic upper limb following stroke is of major concern with only 4–5% of patients regaining function. Numerous traditional treatment approaches are applied in the clinical setting. However, to date very few demonstrate scientific evidence of success.

Bilateral isokinematic training (BIT) is a unique and effective approach to upper limb retraining in 'motor' strokes. It involves the completion of activities using both the affected and the non-affected limb, at the same time, speed and in an identical manner. A hypothetical neurophysiological model underlying the approach has been well established and research conducted in both Melbourne, Australia and Ayrshire, Scotland have demonstrated promising results. Clinical observations also support the effectiveness of this technique, which has enabled patients to achieve significant improvements in upper limb performance in very short periods of time.

Electromyographical biofeedback (sEMG bf) assists therapists' knowledge concerning the degree of control a patient has over muscle action and the kinematic aspects of task performance. Basmajian (1983) defined biofeedback as: 'the technique of using equipment to reveal to human beings some of their subconscious physiologic events, normal and abnormal, in the form of visual and auditory signals, in order to teach them to manipulate these otherwise involuntary or unfelt events, by manipulating the displayed signals'. In this technique, changes in the level of response by a conscious effort to contract or relax muscle groups is fed back to the patient in the form of sensory stimulus. Invariably the stimulus is either auditory, visual or a combination of the two.

Ensuring Best Practice

Occupational Therapy Clinical Audit

The College of Occupational Therapists launched a 'Clinical Audit Information Pack' in 1998. This resource pack was developed by Christine Sealey, Clinical Audit Officer, to assist Occupational Therapists with clinical audit and clinical effectiveness.

The Clinical Audit pack is a very user friendly, yet informative, guide to clinical audit and how it can be used by occupational therapists to evaluate their practice. It comes in A4 ring binder form and includes:

- what is clinical audit and what is clinical effectiveness?;
- audit ideas and examples;
- a simple step-by-step guide to doing audit, including choosing topics, deciding who to involve, selecting methods, setting standards, collecting and analysing data, taking corrective action and re-auditing;
- auditing outcomes with references for commonly used published measures;
- removable laminated audit checklists;
- audit record form (also on disk so you can adapt it to suit yourself);
- information on useful organizations, publications, Internet sites, references and further reading.

> "This is a simple step by step clear guide for OTs new to audit as well as information and methods for those with experience. It made me feel it was something that was possible and desirable for ordinary OTs'.

A copy of the Clinical Audit Information pack can be purchased from the College of Occupational Therapists, 106–114 Borough High Street, Southwark, London SE1 1LB.

The College of Occupational Therapists is planning to launch a database with lists of those doing audits (on any subject) with brief abstracts. This will be available to members.

Occupational Therapy Research

There is limited evidence for the effectiveness of occupational therapy in practice. The following are examples of completed studies that have researched occupational therapy effectiveness:

> Turton A, Fraser C. The use of home therapy programmes for improving recovery of the upper limb following stroke. British Journal of Occupational Therapy 1990; 53(11): 457–62.

The study included 22 patients with residual arm function on discharge from hospital (mean 12 weeks after stroke), 12 received a home therapy programme and 10 received routine care for 8 weeks. Home therapy included a booklet, an individualized programme of exercises, involvement of carers/spouse and a compliance book. Frequency of treatment was 2–3 times every day.

Results indicated that the home therapy group had significantly better scores for the southern motor group's motor assessment, significantly better performance on the ten-hole peg test and compliance rates were high.

Drummond AER, Walker MF. A randomised controlled trial of leisure rehabilitation after stroke. Clinical Rehabilitation 1995; 9: 283–90.

The study included 65 patients discharged from hospital, Group 1 received leisure rehabilitation for 30 minutes a week for 3 months, then 30 minutes a fortnight for 3 months; Group 2 received conventional OT; Group 3 was a control group with no additional input. Outcome measures were gauged at 3 and 6 months.

Results indicated a significant increase in leisure score for group 1 only; this group also had higher mobility scores and showed a trend for improvement in psychological well-being. There was an ongoing multi-centre study, the TOTAL study.

Corr S. Occupational therapy for stroke patients after hospital discharge: a randomised controlled trial. Clinical Rehabilitation 1995; 9: 291–6.

A total of 110 patients were recruited after discharge from two stroke units, 55 in the treatment group and 55 in the control group. Following intervention, the patients were reviewed at 2, 8, 16 and 24 weeks with outcome assessments at one year.

Results indicated no significant differences between the groups for ADL, extended ADL, mood or quality of life. The treatment group received significantly more equipment and the number of hospital readmissions was significantly reduced.

Walker MF, Drummond AER, Lincoln NB. Evaluation of dressing practice for stroke patients after discharge from hospital: a crossover design study. Clinical Rehabilitation 1996; 10: 23–31.

This study included 30 patients with persistent dressing problems 6 months after stroke. Fifteen patients (group 1) received 3 months of intensive dressing practice followed by 3 months of no intervention. The other 15 patients (group 2) received 3 months of no intervention followed by 3 months of intensive dressing practice. They had a mean of seven treatment sessions.

Results indicated a significant increase in dressing abilities for both groups during the treatment phases only, that dressing practice is still effective at 9–12 months after stroke, and that group 1 did not lose their dressing skills after a period of non-intervention.

Clarke PA, Ahern J, Gladman JRF, Lincoln NB. A randomised controlled trial of enhanced social service occupational therapy for stroke patients. Clinical Rehabilitation 1997; 11: 107–13.

From 111 patients recruited, 55 received enhanced service and 58 received routine service with outcome assessments at 3 and 6 months.

Results at 3 months indicated that the enhanced group had received significantly more visits and had higher extended ADL scores. At 6 months there was no significant difference between the groups for extended ADL, but the enhanced group had significantly better mobility scores, and carers of patients receiving the enhanced service were significantly less distressed.

Gilbertson L, Langhorne P, Walker A, Allen A, Murray GD. Domiciliary occupational therapy for patients with stroke discharged from hospital: randomised controlled trial. BMJ, 2000; 320: 603–606

Discharge home would appear to be a critical stage in stroke rehabilitation. Poor coordination of discharge planning, lack of access to services, psychosocial problems and reduced quality of life are a common experience at this time. This randomized controlled trial evaluated the effectiveness of a short post-discharge domiciliary occupational therapy outreach service on the recovery of stroke patients discharged home from hospital. A total of 138 patients were allocated to either a conventional outpatient follow-up group or conventional services plus a six-week domiciliary occupational therapy intervention. All patients were assessed before discharge, at 6 weeks and 6 months to measure functional ability, quality of life, perception of outcome and experience of discharge. Information was also obtained on readmission rates, strain on carers, and resources used to operate the domiciliary service. The data collected provide further information on the potential value of developing domiciliary occupational therapy services for stroke patients discharged home from hospital.

Results indicated that there were no significant demographic differences between the groups at baseline, but at 7 weeks after discharge, the treatment group showed improvements in Barthel ADL index scores and an improvement in patient satisfaction.

Lincoln NB, Husbands S, Trescoli C, Drummond AER, Gladman JRF, Berman P. Five year follow up of a randomised controlled trial of a stroke rehabilitation unit. BMJ, 2000; 320: 549.

Sharon Husbands/Dr Avril Drummond, Ageing and Disability Research Unit, Floor B, Medical School, Queens Medical Centre, Nottingham, NG7 2UH, UK.

The benefits to one year of stroke unit care are well known. Only one study, of a combined acute and rehabilitation unit, has examined the long-term benefit to 5 years. There are no published studies about the long-term benefits of a non-acute stroke rehabilitation unit.

Stroke patients were randomly allocated to care on a stroke rehabilitation unit (SU) ($n = 176$) or care on medical or geriatric wards (CW) ($n = 139$). Patients were followed up at 5 years or until death, by a researcher blind to the initial allocation. The outcome was measured on survival, level of disability, mood and carer strain.

Results at 5 years indicated that 79 (44.9%) of the SU patients and 77 (55.4%) of the CW patients had died; relative risk (RR) on contingency tables = 0.81 (95% CI 0.65–1.01). There were 100 (56.8%) SU patients and 88 (63.3%) CW patients dead or living in care, RR = 0.90 (95% CI 0.75–1.08); 139 (82.3%) SU patients and 114 (90.5%) CW patients were dead or disabled (Barthel 0–18 disabled, 19–20 independent), RR = 0.85 (95% CI 0.72–0.99). Cox's Proportional Hazard Model confirmed that CW patients were more likely to die than SU patients, controlling for age, previous disability and number of vascular risk factors (RR = 0.85; 95% CI 0.72–0.99). Comparison of outcomes in survivors (Mann-Whitney U test) showed no significant differences between the groups in personal and instrumental ADL, mood or adjustment to disability or carer mood.

The conclusion was that the long-term benefits of stroke rehabilitation are due largely to improved survival, and are not negated by the presence of increased residual disability.

Multicentre trial of out-patient occupational therapy for stroke (TOTAL – Trial of Occupational Therapy and Leisure). Does leisure therapy improve outcomes of stroke patients six months after hospital discharge? Presented at Society for Research in Rehabilitation conference 30 June 1999, Sheffield.

Dr Chris Parker/Dr Avril Drummond, Ageing and Disability Research Unit, Floor B, Medical School, Queens Medical Centre, Nottingham NG7 2UH, UK.

The study aimed to evaluate the effectiveness of outpatient occupational therapy, by promoting either independence in ADL ability or participation in leisure studies in reducing disability, increasing leisure participation and improving mood.

Single-centre studies had shown promise with these approaches, but a multicentre trial was required to find out if such an approach was feasible and whether the benefits were generalizable throughout the NHS. A total of

466 patients in five UK centres were included and randomly allocated to three groups. Patients in the two active therapy groups received 10 occupational therapy sessions each, at home, within six months.

Results showed small positive treatment effects but these were not significant.

An exploration of psychological recovery from stroke – a life narrative life approach. Presented at the Occupational Therapy Annual Conference, Liverpool, 22 July 1999.

Dr Caroline Hill, Postdoctoral Research Fellow, University of Southampton, Southampton, UK.

Psychological recovery from stroke was explored using a new perspective, a life-narrative approach. Ten respondents with no prior history of disability gave narrative life interviews in hospital and at home six months and one year following admission for a first-time stroke.

The respondents described a fundamental change in their lives and identity. In hospital, they described a split between their body and who they had been physically and socially. This split appeared to be psychologically distressing and rebuilding this was their main concern over the following year.

Physical impairment had a fundamental psychological and practical effect on the lives of people following a stroke. Occupational therapists should provide social and physical opportunities for stroke survivors to rebuild their body–self relationship during the first year post-stroke.

Walker MF, Gladman JF, Lincoln NB, Siemansma P, Whiteley T. A randomised controlled trial of occupational therapy for stroke patients not admitted to hospital. Lancet 1999; 354 (24 July): 278–80.

Patients who suffer a stroke are not always admitted to hospital. The literature indicates that this group of patients often remains at home with little or no coordinated rehabilitation. Therefore the aim of this study was to evaluate the efficacy of an occupational therapy intervention for stroke patients not admitted to hospital.

Consecutive stroke patients on a community register, one month after stroke, were randomly allocated to an occupational therapy intervention group or to a control group. Patients allocated to the treatment group were treated at home by an occupational therapist for up to five months. Patients were assessed on outcome measures at six months. The main outcome measures used were: Extended Activities of Daily Living (EADL), Barthel ADL index, General Health Questionnaire (GHQ28), Carer Strain Index (CSI) and the London Handicap Scale (LHS) at six months. All assessments were conducted blind by an independent assessor.

Results: 185 patients were included, 94 allocated to the treatment group and 91 to the control group. At follow-up, patients in the treatment group had significantly higher median EADL scores (Mann-Whitney (M-W) $p < 0.01$: estimated difference 3, 95% CI 1 to 4), Barthel ADL scores (M-W $p < 0.01$, difference 1, 95% CI 0 to 1), CSI scores (M-W $p < 0.05$, difference 1, 95% CI 0 to 2) and LHS scores (M-W $p < 0.05$, difference 7, 95% CI 0.3 to 13.5). There were no significant differences in GHQ scores in the patients or carers.

Interpretation: occupational therapy significantly reduced disability and handicap in stroke patients who were not admitted to hospital and also significantly reduced the strain of the carer.

Edmans JA, Webster J, Lincoln NB. A comparison of two approaches in the treatment of perceptual problems in stroke. Clinical Rehabilitation 2000; Vol.14, 250–263..

Perceptual problems are common following stroke and affect the patient's functional ability, suggesting that these problems should be treated.

Eighty patients admitted to the Nottingham Stroke Unit were assessed for perceptual and functional abilities, using standardized assessments (Rivermead Perceptual Assessment Battery and Barthel ADL Index). Each patient identified as having perceptual problems was randomly allocated to one of two groups for perceptual treatment. One followed the transfer of training approach and one followed the functional approach. The study compared the effectiveness of the two approaches in improving perceptual and functional abilities.

Treatment was given for 2.5 hours per week for six weeks. On completion of the six weeks' treatment, each patient was reassessed for perceptual and functional abilities.

The results showed no significant difference between the treatment groups on patient characteristics, or between before and after treatment perceptual total, individual perceptual subtest, or functional total scores (Mann Whitney U 642.5–798.0, $p > 0.05$). Wilcoxon Matched Pairs Signed Ranks Tests showed a significant improvement after treatment, on perceptual and functional abilities, (perceptual $z = 6.02$, $p < 0.001$, functional $z = 6.72$, $p < 0.001$).

These results indicated that the improvement in perceptual abilities was equivalent using either of the two approaches. As this could be spontaneous recovery or due to the effects of the Stroke Unit, a control group of 20 patients was studied. This showed similar results between the treatment groups and controls, suggesting that the improvement was likely to be the effect of being on the Stroke Unit.

Walker MF, Drummond AER, Gatt J, Sackley CM. Occupational therapy treatment for stroke patients: a survey of current practice (submitted for publication).

Despite an increasing body of evidence to support the efficacy of occupational therapy treatment for stroke patients, little is known about the content of therapy administered. Various approaches have been advocated for the treatment of stroke patients in hospital with empirical evidence suggesting that therapists may not just use one approach, but combine different ones depending on their clinical judgement.

A recent survey of physiotherapists demonstrated that although familiar with a wide range of approaches, the most frequently used approach was Bobath. The reason for choosing a particular approach was based on experience gained through practice and not the use of published research results.

The aim of this survey was to examine the practical aspects of stroke care given by Occupational Therapists. Questionnaires, in-depth interviews and case vignettes were used to help explore this issue.

Results: the two most common approaches identified were the functional approach and the Bobath approach. Main indications for choice were age of the patient, progress with other approaches and discharge date. Many occupational therapists were unfamiliar with standardized assessments and were unable to adequately describe the theoretical basis for the treatment used.

Information on *current occupational therapy research projects* is given below. This information was taken from the occupational therapy research register held by the library, at the College of Occupational Therapy, London. Current awareness bulletins about current occupational therapy research are also available from the library, College of Occupational Therapists, London.

Stroke collaborative review group: rehabilitation

Dr Avril Drummond, Ageing and Disability Research Unit, Floor B, Medical School, Queens Medical Centre, Nottingham NG7 2UH, UK.

The Stroke Collaborative Review Group to the Cochrane Collaboration has been established to review all randomized controlled trials of stroke treatment and to perform formal meta-analyses. The rehabilitation reviews are concerned with trials of occupational therapy, speech therapy, cognitive rehabilitation and mood disorders. The process of reviewing stroke rehabilitation trials will involve literature searching of trials in a wide range of neurological conditions and these will also be collated. The aim of this study is to provide a database of randomized controlled trials in rehabilitation to enable meta-analyses and structured overviews to be conducted.

Validation of the Stroke Drivers Screening Assessment (SDSA) for patients with acquired neurological disability

Kate Radford, Stroke Research Unit, Division of Stroke Medicine, City Hospital, Nottingham NG5 1PB, UK.

The assessment of fitness to drive in people suffering from neurological conditions is both time consuming and complex. At present there is little consistency between different centres in the procedures used and conflicting evidence as to which cognitive impairments need to be assessed or which predict driving outcome.

The Stroke Drivers Screening Assessment (SDSA) is a collection of three cognitive tests which have been found to be predictive of driving ability in stroke patients. The purpose of this study is to determine whether SDSA is predictive of driving ability in patients with other acquired neurological conditions such as head injury, multiple sclerosis etc. A total of 150 people referred to Derby Regional Mobility Centre for assessment of their fitness to drive will be assessed on the SDSA. An independent assessment of the individual's driving ability will be carried out by a driving instructor who will make the decision about his/her fitness to drive. The prediction of fitness to drive from the SDSA will be compared with the decision made at the Derby Regional Mobility Centre. This will indicate whether the SDSA can be used as a screening assessment for patients with acquired neurological disability.

The contribution of reorganized motor pathways to recovery of arm and hand function after stroke

Ailie Turton, Eastfields, Littleton-on-Severn, Bristol BS12 1NS, UK.

Stroke often disrupts the descending motor pathways controlling the upper limb with severe consequences for the patient's hand function. Although some recover they are often slow and clumsy when using the affected hand. The mechanism underlying recovery is an unsettled question. Transcranial magnetic stimulation (TMS) was used to determine the changes in the connectivity and function of the corticospinal tract (CST) that are associated with improved motor performance in the recovering arm and hand. The study comprised four parts:

1. Task dependency of responses to TMS in recovered stroke patients: eight patients who had recovered some degree of hand function were tested for task dependence of short-latency EMG responses to TMS. Normal subjects were also tested.
2. Longitudinal investigation of recovery of voluntary movement of arm and hand after stroke: the relationship between the recovery of hand and arm function in a group of acute stroke patients ($n = 21$) and the presence of short latency contralateral and ipsilateral EMG responses to TMS in four difference upper limb muscles were investigated.

3. Ipsilateral responses in normal subjects: the results of the longitudinal study prompted further investigation of the presence of ipsilateral responses in proximal and distal muscles in 15 normal subjects.

4. The contribution of CS input to production of force in proximal and distal upper limb muscles: because patients did not always have responses to TMS in recovered proximal muscles, two further studies were carried out to clarify the contribution of CS input to production of force in proximal and distal upper limb muscles.

A survey of rehabilitation in nursing homes in Nottingham

Marion Walker, Stroke Research Unit, Division of Stroke Medicine, City Hospital, Nottingham NG5 1PB, UK.

There have been several studies documenting the rehabilitation needs of stroke patients in hospital and in the community, but unfortunately little is known about the rehabilitation needs of stroke patients in nursing homes. Through work with stroke patients in the community it has been noticed that the availability of rehabilitation in nursing homes is very variable. Some nursing homes finance their own physiotherapists and activity/occupational therapists but the policy for financing such rehabilitation seems unclear. It would appear that there is some inequity in accessing care for residents in nursing homes.

The aims of this survey are to record the level of rehabilitation activity in nursing homes in Nottingham, how rehabilitation is accessed and how it is financed. In-depth interviews will be used to explore the content of treatment provided by occupational therapists and physiotherapists.

The Stroke Association centenary home therapy project

Margaret Goose, Chief Executive, Stroke Association, London, UK.

This project is designed to pilot a new model in the North East of England, namely that if a stroke patient was accompanied home by a therapist, who would work with him/her during prolonged daily visits for a period of up to eight weeks, he/she would gain confidence and achieve goals that he/she would not otherwise have done. In meeting any problem posed by the home environment, the patient's and carer's confidence would be boosted by the knowledge that expert help and advice were at hand.

Three teams will be recruited in three different locations, each team consisting of an occupational therapist and two occupational therapy assistants. In collaboration with participating hospitals, each stroke patient will be assessed prior to discharge. The patient will be offered a list of goals that he/she might wish to achieve in three areas: personal care, domestic chores and social activities. The goals are those that give the patient confidence, dignity and independence in life after stroke and will be agreed by the patient with the therapist in order of priority.

The occupational therapy team will work with the patient, accompanying him/her at the time of discharge and remaining with the patient and carer for a significant part of the first day at home. Subsequent visits will be as often and for as long as required, up to a maximum of eight weeks, to enable the patient to achieve the agreed goals. The patient will be assessed during this period and again at six months, using nationally agreed measurements.

The project will continue at each of the three sites for two years, and will be monitored continuously and evaluated by an independent auditor, in agreement with the local NHS and Social Services. During this period it is planned that each team will assist over 200 patients. It was aimed to recruit staff by June 1999, to develop policies, procedures and processes, and to be ready to commence the service in September 1999. The anticipated costs are £150 000 per team over the two and a half years of the project i.e. £450 000 in total.

Competency Framework

A competency framework for clinical, managerial and behavioural competency models has been developed by the Occupational Therapy Department at Queens Medical Centre in Nottingham. Their ideas and methods are described below.

All individuals deserve to know what is expected of them in terms of the role they are performing, the level to which they are expected to perform, to be given guidance and support for areas where their performance needs to improve and to have a vision of their own career, next possible steps and what it will take to achieve them.

Competences are a combination of the relevant job knowledge, skills and behaviours needed to undertake a role to the specified standard.

Having such an approach is a positive way of ensuring that staff receive the necessary training and/or development to meet service objectives. Training is therefore targeted to the skills, knowledge or behaviours required in a particular role. Using this process, both the individual and his/her supervisor are much clearer about each other's expectations and the priorities.

What are the Benefits?

Benefits include:

* bringing out the best in staff to meet service objectives;
* increasing effectiveness;
* improving quality of care;

- acknowledging the contribution of each individual;
- helping each individual understand his/her contribution to the success of a service or organization;
- helping staff understand what is expected of them;
- developing a sharp focus for supervision and appraisal;
- helping staff at all levels – whether supervisor or supervisee – understand about the differing expectations in each grade of post.

Where to Begin

It is important to bear in mind the following:

- To achieve compliance, involve staff early. They will feel empowered if they develop the competences in small groups.
- In order to develop a competency-based approach to practice, you will need a robust supervision and appraisal process.
- Enthusiasm is required to complete the process. It does take a long time.
- Do not be tempted to take a framework and apply it directly to yourself, your staff or your service. Competency frameworks are effective when they are tailored to local requirements. By all means use the basis of styles of documentation used elsewhere, but develop your own for your specific needs.

Helpful Hints

- The process will not be successful if the manager is not committed or is not prepared to spend the necessary time needed.
- Staff need to clearly understand the benefits.
- Clear service objectives are needed so that roles and posts are well defined.
- When objectives are set, whether they are individual, team or service, they should be SMART:
  S   –   specific;
  M   –   measurable;
  A   –   achievable;
  R   –   realistic;
  T   –   timely.
- Any competences must reflect the culture of the service or organization and must be regularly updated to reflect current need.

Individual Competences

Each competency should comprise:

- key role/tasks;
- competence level required;

- development required/achieved;
- method for achievement.

Example of a Basic-grade Clinical Competency

(a) *Key role*: To assess occupational performance and plan and carry out goal-orientated rehabilitation programmes.
(b) *Competence level required*: An understanding of the theory of occupational therapy. The ability to implement the occupational therapy process with appropriate supervision:
  - gather/evaluate information;
  - prioritize allocated caseload;
  - identify problems/goals;
  - develop a treatment programme;
  - implement a treatment programme;
  - review, reassess and evaluate progress;
  - discharge planning.
(c) *Development required/achieved*:
  - development of clinical skills and knowledge;
  - ability and confidence in managing caseload.
(d) *Method of achievement*:
  - gained through ongoing clinical experience;
  - discussion and guidance from senior therapist;
  - observation of senior staff;
  - training specific to individual areas including team teaching, inservice teaching, condition-specific lectures and seminars;
  - develop self-directed learning including reading, journal reviews, literature searches.

Behavioural Competency Model

Introduction

There are four units of competence identified in the behavioural competency model against which individuals self-evaluate prior to an annual appraisal of a planned supervision session:

- Unit A – managing yourself;
- Unit B – enabling and motivating others;
- Unit C – working to achieve success;
- Unit D – decision making.

The competency model is aimed at encouraging self-awareness, self-development and improving effectiveness. The process is intended to be non-threatening, constructive and handled with a 'no blame' culture. It is essential that good performance is acknowledged and that staff having difficulty are given feedback and training and development opportunities.

Competency Framework Policy and Procedure

Introduction

1.1. Staff are our most valuable asset, providing a creative, flexible and professional service.

1.2. The individual contribution and performance of each member of staff is valued regardless of experience, grade or perceived status.

1.3. The competency framework aims to help staff understand what is expected of them, encourage self-evaluation in attitudes, behaviours, skills and abilities, and work towards setting and maintaining high standards in all areas of work.

1.4. The competency framework acknowledges good practice and facilitates the identification of training needs for further personal and professional development.

Policy

The competency framework comprises a range of clinical and/or managerial competency models for all grades of staff. In addition there is a behavioural model which utilizes a self-assessment questionnaire:

2.1. The competency framework will be used as follows:

2.1.1. To assist in the supervision process formally and informally throughout the year.

2.1.2. With a new member of staff to help identify the training and development required.

2.1.3. When a current member of staff is promoted or appointed to a new post.

2.1.4. Six-monthly with rotational basic grade staff.

2.1.5. With all staff annually prior to the appraisal and objective-setting process.

2.2. Information gained or issues discussed will remain confidential between the supervisor and supervisee and will be used in a creative manner. Only where there is concern that an individual is unsafe or considered not competent to practise should issues be discussed with the manager and/or deputy.

2.3. Timescales will be as follows:

2.3.1. With new staff members, regraded staff or basic grade rotational staff, within one month of starting work.

2.3.2. With all staff at the annual appraisal and objective setting session. Staff will be asked to self-evaluate against the competency models not more than two weeks prior to the date set. A personal development plan will be agreed after the appraisal.

2.4. Adequate time will be set aside by the supervisor and supervisee with guaranteed privacy. Bleeps and pagers will be left with other team members or at reception and an interruption-free policy will be adhered to.

Procedure

3.1. A mutually agreed time and date will be set by the supervisor and supervisee.

3.2. The supervisee will be issued with the appropriate paperwork prior to the date.

3.3. Discussion between the supervisor and supervisee in the meeting should be open, honest, not defensive and in a 'no blame' culture.

3.4. It is expected that the supervisor and supervisee will illustrate each element with examples of behaviours, attitudes, skills and abilities.

3.5. Elements in the models may be regarded as 'not seen' or 'not applicable' with the agreement of both parties.

3.6. The agreed objectives will be monitored and reviewed within the regular supervision sessions.

3.7. Once complete, the paperwork will be placed in personal files. Individuals may take a photocopy if desired.

Full details about this competency framework can be obtained by contacting Patricia Church, Head OT, OT Department, Queens Medical Centre, Nottingham NG7 2UH.

Glossary

Agnosia: Inability to recognize familiar objects perceived by the senses.

Ataxia: Loss of coordination and smooth interplay between muscles in the cerebellum due to damage leading to uncontrolled jerky movement.

Cognition: The ability to use and integrate basic capacities such as perception, language memory and thought.

Contracture: Shortening of soft tissues within the joint due to abnormal tonal changes and prolonged positioning in a fixed posture.

Dysarthria: Weakness or incoordination of the speech muscles that prevents clear pronunciation of words.

Dysphagia: Difficulty in swallowing.

Dysphasia: Difficulty understanding language and/or expressing self as a result of a brain injury.

Dyspraxia: Inability to perform certain skilled purposeful movements despite having intact the relevant motor, sensory and coordination functions.

Dystonia: Asymmetry of involuntary contracting muscles resulting in unusual contortions of the body.

Flaccidity: Absence of normal tension (tone) in the muscles.

Hemianopia: Damage to the part of the brain that interprets visual information, resulting in blindness of part of the visual field, although the patient's eyes and optic tracts are undamaged.

Hemiplegia: Paralysis affecting one side of the body.

Heterotrophic ossification: Appearance of bone in soft tissues, often occurring in large joints, i.e. elbow, knee, ankle, in patients with severe brain injury and prolonged unconsciousness.

Ideational apraxia: Inability to carry out activities automatically or on command because the patient no longer understands the idea or concept of the task.

Ideomotor apraxia: Inability to initiate gestures or perform purposeful motor tasks on command even though the patient fully understands the concept or idea of the task.

151

Lability: Decreased ability to moderate the expression of emotion, e.g. person might burst into tears without feeling sad, or may laugh inappropriately in an upsetting situation.

Perception: The process by which we organize and interpret patterns of stimuli (e.g. visual, auditory, tactile) in the environment.

Perseveration: Continued repetition of movement, word or idea.

Proprioception: The ability to judge movements in the joints of the body.

Spasticity: More than normal muscle tension (tone).

Stereognosis: The ability to identify objects by touch.

Unilateral neglect (inattention): Inability to integrate and use perceptions from the left side of the body or the left side of the environment.

References

Agrell B, Dehlin O. Comparison of six depression rating scales in geriatric stroke patients. Stroke 1989; 20: 1190–4.

Aho K, Harmsen P, Hatano S, Marquardsen J, Smirnov VE, Strasser T. Cerebrovascular disease in the community: sesults of a WHO collaborative study. Bulletin of the World Health Organisation 1980; 58 (1): 113–30.

Allen LR, Beattie RU. The role of leisure as an indicator of overall satisfaction with community life. Journal of Leisure Research 1984; 2: 99–109.

Anderson E, Choy E. Parietal lobe syndromes in hemiplegia, a program for treatment. American Journal of Occupational Therapy 1970; 24: 13–18.

Ayres AJ. Sensory Integration and Learning Disorders. Los Angeles: Western Psychological Services, 1980.

Badley EM. Measurement and revision of the ICIDH. Paper presented at British Society of Rehabilitation Medicine and Society for Research in Rehabilitation summer meeting, University of Leeds, 1997.

Bamford J. 'Is it a stroke and what sort of a stroke is it?' Hospital Update 1991; November: 891–6.

Basmajian JV. Reflex cervical muscle spasm: treatment by diazepam, phenobarbital or placebo. Archives of Physical Medicine and Rehabilitation 1983; 64(3): 121–4.

Basmajian JV, Gowland CA, Finlayson AJ, Hall AL, Swanson LR, Stratford PW et al. Stroke treatment: comparison of integrated behavioural-physical therapy vs. traditional physical therapy programs. Archives of Physical Medicine and Rehabilitation 1987; 68: 267–72.

Bassetlaw Physiotherapy Research Group, 1992. The POEM Catalogue. Contact the Physiotherapy Adviser, Bassetlaw Hospital and Community Services NHS Trust. Tel: 01909 500990.

Benjamin J. The Northwick Park ADL Index. British Journal of Occupational Therapy 1976; 39(12): 301–6.

Bennett-Levy J, Powell GE. The Subjective Memory Questionnaire: an investigation into the self-reporting of 'real-life' memory skills. British Journal of Social and Clinical Psychology 1980; 19: 177–88.

Benton AL, Hamsher K de S. Multilingual Aphasia Examination. Test Manual. Iowa City: AJA Associates, 1989.

Bobath B. Adult Hemiplegia: Evaluation and Treatment. London: Heinemann, 1976.

Bobath B. Adult Hemiplegia: Evaluation and Treatment, 3rd edn. London: Heinemann, 1990.

Boehme R. Improving Upper Body Control. USA: Psychological Corporation, 1995.

Bower E. Physiotherapy for cerebral palsy: a historical review. Bailliere's Clinical Neurology 1993; 2(1): 29–54.

Brunnstrom S. Movement Therapy in Hemiplegia. London: Harper & Row, 1970.

Burgess I, Pearce M, Lincoln NB, Dean M. The Salford Objective Recognition Test. Nottingham: Nottingham Rehab, 1994.

Burgess PW, Shallice T. The Hayling and Brixton Tests. Bury St Edmunds: Thames Valley Test Company, 1997.

Burt M. Perceptual deficits in hemiplegia. American Journal of Nursing 1970; 70: 1026–9.

Carey LM. Somatosensory loss after stroke. Physical Rehabilitation Medicine 1995; 7(1): 51–91.

Carr EK, Lincoln NB. Inter-rater reliability of the Rey figure copying test. British Journal of Clinical Psychology 1988; 27: 267–8.

Carr JH, Shepherd RB. A Motor Relearning Programme for Stroke, 2nd edn. London: Heinemann Physiotherapy, 1987.

Collin C, Wade DT, Davis S, Home V. The Barthel ADL Index: a reliability study. International Disability Studies 1988; 10(2): 61–3.

Cook S, Spreadbury P. Trent Occupational Therapy Clinical Audit and Outcomes Project. Trent Regional Health Authority, 1995 [available from COT].

Coppard BM, Lohman H. Introduction to Splinting – A Critical Thinking and Problem-solving Approach. St Louis, MO: Mosby, 1996.

Davies PM. Steps to Follow. New York: Springer-Verlag, 1985.

DeSouza LH. The effects of sensation and motivation on regaining movement control following stroke. Physiotherapy 1983; 69(7): 238–40.

Dickstein R, Hocherman S, Pillar T, Shaham R. Stroke rehabilitation: three exercise therapy approaches. Physical Therapy 1986; 66(8): 1233–8.

Diller L, Gordon W. Interventions for cognitive deficits in brain-injured adults. Journal of Consulting and Clinical Psychology 1981; 49(6): 822–34.

Diller L, Weinberg J. Hemi-inattention in rehabilitation: the evolution of a rational remediation program. Advances in Neurology 1977; 18: 63–82.

Drummond AER. Leisure activity after stroke. International Disability Studies 1990; 12: 157–60.

Drummond AER, Walker MF. A randomised controlled trial of leisure rehabilitation after stroke. Clinical Rehabilitation 1995; 9: 283–90.

Drummond AER, Walker MF. The Nottingham leisure questionnaire for stroke patients. British Journal of Occupational Therapy 1994; 57: 414–18.

Duff JD, Campbell JJ. The regional prefrontal syndrome: a theoretical and clinical overview. Journal of Neuropsychiatry 1994; 8 (4): 379–87.

Eakin P. Assessments of activities of daily living: a critical review. British Journal of Occupational Therapy 1989a; 52 (1): 11–15.

Eakin P. Problems with assessments of activities of daily living. British Journal of Occupational Therapy, 1989b; 52 (2): 50–4.

Ebrahim S, Barer D, Nouri F. Affective illness after stroke. British Journal of Psychiatry 1987; 151: 52–6.

Ebrahim S, Noun FM, Barer D. Measuring disability after a stroke. Journal of Epidemiology and Community Health 1985; 39: 86–9.

Edmans JA. An investigation of stroke patients resuming sexual activity. British Journal of Occupational Therapy 1998; 61 (1): 36–8.

Edmans JA, Goodwin N, Foster A, O'Reilly M, Stout E. The development of a care pathway for stroke rehabilitation. British Journal of Therapy and Rehabilitation 1997; 4(10): 559–62.

Edmans JA, Webster J. The Edmans ADL index: validity and reliability. Disability and Rehabilitation 1997; 19(11): 465–76.

Edwards S. Neurological Physiotherapy: a Problem Solving Approach. London: Churchill Livingstone, 1996.

Ernst E. A review of stroke rehabilitation and physiotherapy. Stroke 1990; 21(7): 1081–5.

Fisher AG. Assessment of Motor and Process Skills. Fort Collins, CO: Three Star Press, 1999.

Garratt AM, Ruta DA, Abdulla MI, Buckingham JK, Russell IT. The SF 36 health survey questionnaire: an outcome measure suitable for routine use within the NHS? British Medical Journal 1993; 306(6890): 1440–4.

Goff B. Appropriate afferent stimulation. Physiotherapy 1969; 55: 9–17.

Goldberg DP, Hiller VF. A scaled version of the general health questionnaire. Physiology and Medicine 1979; 9: 139–45.

Golding E. The Middlesex Elderly Assessment of Mental State. Bury St Edmunds: Thames Valley Test Company, 1989.

Granger CV, Albrecht GL, Hamilton BB. Outcome of comprehensive medical rehabilitation: measurement by PULSES profile and Barthel index. Archives of Physical Medicine and Rehabilitation 1979; 60: 145–54.

Granger CV, Hamilton BB, Sherwin FS. Guide for the Use of the Uniform Data Set for Medical Rehabilitation. New York: Uniform Data System for Medical Rehabilitation Project Office [Buffalo General Hospital, New York 14203, USA] 1986.

Greveson G, James O. Improving long-term outcome after stroke – the views of patients and carers. Health Trends 1991; 23: 161–2.

Grieve E. The stroke patient as a person: body-image and sexuality. In Harrison MA. Physiotherapy in Stroke Management. Edinburgh: Churchill Livingstone, 1995.

Hagedorn R. Occupational Therapy: Foundations for Practice. London: Churchill Livingstone, 1992.

Hanger HC, Walker G, Paterson LA, McBride S, Sainsbury R. What do patients and their carers want to know about stroke? A two-year follow-up study. Clinical Rehabilitation 1998; 12: 45–52.

Harrison MA. Physiotherapy in Stroke Management London: Churchill Livingstone, 1995.

Hecaen H, Assal G. A comparison of constructive deficits following right and left hemispheric lesions. Neuropsychologia 1970; 8: 289–303.

Holbrook M, Skilbeck CE. An activities index for use with stroke patients. Age and Ageing 1983; 12: 166–70.

Itzkovich M, Elazar B, Averbuch S. Loewenstein Occupational Therapy Cognitive Assessment, Pequannock, NJ: Maddok, 1993.

Jackson T. Dyspraxia: guidelines for intervention. British Journal of Occupational Therapy 1999; 62 (7): 321–6.

Johnstone M. Home care for the stroke patient: living in a pattern. Edinburgh: Churchill Livingstone, 1980.

Katz S, Ford AB, Moskowitz RW, Jackson BA, Jaffe MW. Studies of illness in the aged. The index of ADL: a standardised measure of biological and psychological function. Journal of the American Medical Association 1963; 185: 914–19.

Kay T. Minor Head Injury: Introduction for professionals. Framingham, MA: National Head Injury Foundation, 1986.

Kertesz A, Ferro JM. Lesion size and location in ideomotor apraxia. Brain 1984; 107: 921–33.

Kidd G, Lawes N, Musa I. A Critical Review of Contemporary Theories. Understanding Neuromuscular Plasticity: A Basis for Clinical Rehabilitation. London: Edward Arnold, 1992.

Kielhofner G (Ed). A Model of Human Occupations. Baltimore, MD: Williams & Wilkins, 1985.

Kinsella GJ, Duffy FD. Psychological readjustment in the spouses of aphasic patients. Scandinavian Journal of Rehabilitation Medicine 1979; 11: 129–32.

Kinsman R. A conductive education approach to stroke patients at Barnet General Hospital. Physiotherapy 1989; 75(7): 418–21.

Kinsman R, Verity R, Waller J. A conductive education approach for adults with neurological dysfunction. Physiotherapy 1988; 74(5): 277–80.

Knott M, Voss D. Proprioceptive Neuromuscular Facilitation, 2nd edn. London: Harper & Row, 1968.

Labi MLC, Phillips TF, Gresham GE. Psycholosocial disability in physically restored long term stroke survivors. Archives of Physical Medicine and Rehabilitation 1980; 61: 561–5.

Laidler P. Stroke Rehabilitation – Structure and Strategy. London: Chapman & Hall, 1994.

Langlois S, MacKinnon JR, Pederson L. Hand splints and cerebral spasticity: a review of the literature. Canadian Journal of Occupational Therapy 1989; 56: 113–19.

Law M, Baptiste S, Carswell-Opzoomer A, McCall M, Polatajko H, Pollock N. Canadian Occupational Performance Measure. Toronto: CAOT Publications ACE, 1991.

Le Roux A. TELER: the concept. Physiotherapy 1993; 79(11): 755–8.

Lezak MD. The problem of assessing executive functions. International Journal of Psychology 1982; 17: 281–97.

Lezak MD. Newer contributions to the neuropsychological assessment of executive functions. Journal of Head Trauma Rehabilitation 1993; March: 24–31.

Lezak MD. Neuropsychological Assessment. Oxford University Press, 1995.

Liepmann H. Uber Störungen des Handelns bei Gehirnkranken. Berlin: Karger, 1905.

Lincoln NB, Crow JL, Jackson JM, Waters GR, Adams SA, Hodgson P. The unreliability of sensory assessments. Clinical Rehabilitation 1991; 5: 272–82.

Lincoln NB, Drummond AER, Edmans JA, Yeo D, Willis D. The Rey figure copy as a screening instrument for perceptual deficits after stroke. British Journal of Occupational Therapy 1998; 61(1): 33–5.

Lincoln NB, Edmans JA. A shortened version of the Rivermead Perceptual Assessment Battery? Clinical Rehabilitation 1989; 3: 199–204.

Lincoln NB, Edmans JA. A re-validation of the Rivermead ADL scale for elderly patients with stroke. Age and Ageing 1990; 19: 19–24.

Lincoln NB, Gamlen R, Thomason H. Behavioural mapping of patients on a stroke unit. International Disability Studies 1989; 11: 149–54.

Logigian MK, Samuels MA, Falconer J, Zagar R. Clinical exercise trial for stroke patients. Archives of Physical Medicine and Rehabilitation 1983; 64(August): 364–7.

Lord J, Hall K. Neuromuscular reeducation versus traditional programs for stroke rehabilitation. Archives of Physical Medicine and Rehabilitation 1986; 67(February): 88–91.

Luria AR. Higher Cortical Functions in Man. New York: Basic Books, 1966.

Lynch M, Grisogono V. Strokes and Head Injuries: A Guide for Patients, Families, Friends and Carers. London: John Murray, 1991.

Mahoney FI, Barthel DW. Functional evaluation: The Barthel Index. Maryland State Medical Journal 1965; February: 61–3.

Malia K, Brannagan A. Cognitive Rehabilitation Workshop 1997.

Mancini JA. Leisure satisfaction and psychological well being in old age: effects of age and outcome. Journal of the American Geriatric Society 1978; 26(12): 550–2.

Miller N. Dyspraxia and its Management. Beckenham: Croom Helm, 1986.

Mosey AC. Occupational Therapy: Configuration of a Profession. New York: Raven Press, 1981.

Mulley GP. Practical Stroke Management. London: Chapman & Hall, 1985.

Nelson HE. A modified card sorting test sensitive to frontal lobe defects. Cortex 1976; 12: 313–324.

Norman DA. Categorisation of action slips. Psychological Review 1981; 88: 1–15.

Nouri FM, Lincoln NB. An extended ADL scale for stroke patients. Clinical Rehabilitation 1987; 1: 301–5.

Nouri FM, Lincoln NB. Stroke Drivers Screening Assessment. Nottingham: Nottingham Rehab, 1994.

Nouri FM, Tinson DJ, Lincoln NB. Cognitive ability and driving after stroke. International Disability Studies 1987; 9: 110–15.

Ottenbacher J, Cusick A. Goal attainment scaling as a method of clinical evaluation. American Journal of Occupational Therapy 1990; 44, 6: 519–25.

Parker CJ, Gladman JRF, Drummond AER et al. A multi-centre randomised controlled trial of leisure therapy and conventional occupational therapy after stroke. Submitted for publication, 1999.

Pigott R, Brickett F. Visual neglect. American Journal of Nursing 1966; 66: 101–5.

Powell T. Head Injury: A Practical Guide. Bicester: Winslow Press, 1994.

Raven JC. Guide to Using the Coloured Progressive Matrices. London: Lewis, 1958.

Reed KL. Models of Practice in Occupational Therapy. Baltimore, MD: Williams & Wilkins, 1984.

Rey A. Le teste de copie de figure complexe. Paris: Editions Centre de Psychologie Appliquée, 1959.

Robertson IH, Gray JM, McKenzie S. Microcomputer based cognitive rehabilitation of visual neglect: three multiple-baseline single case studies. Brain Injury 1988; 2: 151–63.

Robertson IH, Ward T, Ridgeway V, Nimmo-Smith I. The Test of Everyday Attention. Bury St Edmunds: Thames Valley Test Company, 1994.

Robinson RG, Kubos K, Starr LB, Price TR. A two year longitudinal study of post-stroke mood disorders: findings during the initial evaluation. Stroke 1983; 14: 736–41.

Robinson RG, Starr LB, Price TR. A two year longitudinal study of mood disorders following stroke: prevalence and duration at six months follow up. British Journal of Psychiatry 1984; 144: 256–62.

Royal College of Physicians. National Clinical Guidelines for Stroke. London: Royal College of Physicians Publications Unit, 2000.

Sanderson S, Reed KL. Concepts of Occupational Therapy. Baltimore, MD: Williams & Wilkins, 1980.

Sawner K, LaVigne J. Brunnstrom's Movement Therapy in Hemiplegia: A Neurophysiological Approach, 2nd edn. Philadelphia: Lippincott, 1992.

Schmidt RA. A schema theory of discrete motor skill learning. Psychological Review 1975; 82: 225–60.

Schoening HA, Anderegg L, Bergstrom D, Fonda M, Steinke N, Ulrich P. Numerical scoring of self care status of patients. Archives of Physical Medicine and Rehabilitation 1965; 46: 689–97.

Shallice T, Evans ME. The involvement of the frontal lobes in cognitive estimation. Cortex 1978; 14: 294–303.

Sheikh K, Smith DS, Meade TW, Goldenberg E, Brennan PJ, Kinsella G. Repeatability and validity of a modified ADL index of chronic disability. International Rehabilitation Medicine 1979; 1(2): 51–8.

Siev E, Freishtat B. Perceptual dysfunction in the adult stroke patient. New Jersey: Slack, 1976.

Sinyor D, Amato P, Kaloupek DG, Becker R, Goldenberg M, Coopersmith H. Post-stroke depression: relationships to functional impairment, copying strategies and rehabilitation outcome. Stroke 1986; 17(6): 1102–7.

Sjogren K. Leisure after stroke. International Rehabilitation Medicine 1982; 4: 80–7.

Smith ME. The Edinburgh Stroke rehabilitation study. British Journal of Occupational Therapy 1979; 42(6): 139–42.

Snaith RP, Ahmed SN, Mehta S, Hamilton M. Assessments of the severity of primary depressive illness. Psychological Medicine 1971; 1: 143–9.

Sneegas JJ. Components of life satisfaction in middle and later life adults: perceived social competence, leisure participation and leisure satisfaction. Journal of Leisure Research 1986; 20: 17–24.

Sohlberg MM, Mateer CA, Stuss D. Contemporary approaches to the management of executive control dysfunction. Journal of Head Trauma Rehabilitation 1993; March: 45–58.

Spencer C, Clark M, Smith DS. A modification of the Northwick Park ADL Index (the Australian ADL Index). British Journal of Occupational Therapy 1986; 49(11): 350–3.

Stuss DT, Benson DF. The frontal lobes and control of cognition and memory. In Perecman E (Ed). The Frontal Lobes Revisited. New York: IRBN, 1987.

Sullivan P, Markos P, Minor M. An integrated approach to therapeutic exercise. Reston, VA: 1982. Cited in Harrison MA. Physiotherapy in Stroke Management. London: Churchill Livingstone, 1995.

Tate RL, McDonald S. What is apraxia? The clinician's dilemma. Neuropsychological Rehabilitation 1995; 5(4): 273–97.

Taylor MM. Controlled evaluation of percept-concept-motor training therapy after stroke resulting in left hemiplegia. Research grant RD-2215-M, sponsored by Rehabilitation Institute, Detroit: September 1969.

Testani-Dufour L, Marano Morrison CA. Brain attack: correlative anatomy. Journal of Neuroscience Nursing 1997; 29(4): 213–23.

Tyerman R, Tyerman A, Howard P, Hadfield C. Chessington Occupational Therapy Neurological Assessment Battery. Nottingham: Nottingham Rehab, 1986.

Van Heugten CM, Dekker J, Stehmann-Saris JC, Kinebanian A. Empirical Evaluation of OT Protocol for CVA Patients with Apraxia. Utrecht: The Netherlands Institute of Primary Care and The Netherlands School for OT. (Unpublished)

Wade DT. Stroke, Practical Guides for General Practice 4. Oxford: Oxford University Press, 1988.

Wade DT. Measurement in Neurological Rehabilitation. Oxford: Oxford University Press, 1992.

Wade DT, Legh-Smith J, Hewer RL. Social activities after stroke. International Rehabilitation Medicine 1985; 7(4): 176–81.

Warrington E. Recognition Memory Test. Windsor: NFER-Nelson, 1984.

Warrington E, James M. Visual Object and Space Perception Battery. Bury St Edmunds: Thames Valley Test Company, 1991.

Wechsler D. The Wechsler Adult Intelligence Scale Manual. New York: Psychological Corporation, 1955.

Wechsler D. Wechsler Memory Scale Revised. Test Manual. San Antonio, TX: Psychological Corporation, 1987.

Wellwood I, Dennis MS, Warlow CP. Perceptions and knowledge of stroke among surviving patients with stroke and their carers. Age and Ageing 1994; 23(4): 293–8.

Whiting SE, Lincoln NB. An ADL assessment for stroke patients. British Journal of Occupational Therapy 1980; 43(2): 44–6.

Whiting S, Lincoln NB, Bhavnani G, Cockburn J. The Rivermead Perceptual Assessment Battery. Windsor: NFER-Nelson, 1985.

Wilson BA, Alderman N, Burgess P, Emslie H, Evans JJ. Behavioural Assessment of the Dysexecutive Syndrome. Bury St Edmunds: Thames Valley Test Company, 1996.

Wilson BA, Cockburn J, Baddeley A. The Rivermead Behavioural Memory Test. Bury St Edmunds: Thames Valley Test Company, 1985.

Wilson BA, Cockburn J, Halligan P. Behavioural Inattention Test. Bury St Edmunds: Thames Valley Test Company, 1987.

Winward CE, Halligan PW, Wade DT. Rivermead Assessment of Somatosensory Performance. Bury St Edmunds: Thames Valley Test Company, 2000.

Ylvisaker M, Prigatano GP [1987]. Cited in Ylvisaker M, Szekeres SF. Metacognitive and executive impairments in head injured children and adults. Topics in Language Disorders 1989; 9(2): 34–49.

Ylvisaker M, Szekeres SF. Metacognitive and executive impairments in head injured children and adults. Topics in Language Disorders 1989; 9(2): 34–49.

Youngson RM. Stroke: A Self-help Manual for Stroke Sufferers and their Relatives. Devon: David & Charles, 1987.

Zigmond AS, Snaith RP. The hospital anxiety and depression scale. Acta Psychiatrica Scandinavica 1983; 67: 361–70.

Zoltan B. Vision, Perception and Cognition: A Manual for the Evaluation and Treatment of the Neurologically Impaired Adult. New Jersey: Slack, 1996.

Zoltan B, Siev E, Freishtat B. The Adult Stroke Patient: A Manual for Evaluation and Treatment of Perceptual and Cognitive Dysfunction. New Jersey: Slack, 1986.

Useful Books

Ada L, Canning C. Key Issues in Neurological Physiotherapy. London: Heinemann Medical, 1990. ISBN 07 506 000 98.

Allen CMC, Harrison MJG, Wade DT. The Management of Acute Stroke. Tunbridge Wells: Castle House Publications, 1988. ISBN 0 7194 0122 4.

Bickerstaff E. Neurology. London: Edward Arnold, 1989. ISBN 0 340 39487 0.

Bobath B. Abnormal Postural Reflex Activity Caused by Brain Lesions. Oxford: Heinemann Medical, 1986. ISBN 0 433 03300 2.

Bobath B. Adult Hemiplegia: Evaluation and Treatment. Oxford: Heinemann Medical, 1978. ISBN 0 433 03334 7.

Boehme R. Improving Upper Body Control. New York: Psychological Corporation, 1995. ISBN 0 7616 4137 8.

Carr J, Shepherd R. A Motor Relearning Programme for Stroke. London: Heinemann Physiotherapy, 1987. ISBN 0 433 05152 3.

Cohen H. Neuroscience for Rehabilitation. Philadelphia/Baltimore: Lippincott Williams & Wilkins, 1999. ISBN 0 397 55465 6.

Cotton E, Kinsman R. Conductive Education for Adult Hemiplegia. Edinburgh: Churchill Livingstone, 1983. ISBN 0 443 02723 4.

Crombie I. Pocket Guide to Critical Appraisal. London: BMJ Publishing Group, 1998. ISBN 0 7279 1099 X.

Dardier E. The Early Stroke Patient. London: Bailliere Tindall, 1980. ISBN 0 7020 0729 3.

Davies PM. Right in the Middle. Berlin: Springer-Verlag, 1990. ISBN 3 540 51242 X/0 387 51242 X.

Davies PM. Starting Again. Berlin: Springer-Verlag, 1994. ISBN 3 540 55934 5/0 387 55934 5.

Davies PM. Steps to Follow. Berlin: Springer-Verlag, 1985. ISBN 3 540 13436 0/0 387 13436 0.

Demyer W. Neuroanatomy. Chichester: Wiley, 1988. ISBN 0 471 82923 4.

Diamond MC, Scheibel AB, Elson LM. Human Brain Colouring Book. London: Harper Perennial, 1985. ISBN 0 06 460306 7.

Downie PA. Cash's Textbook of Neurology for Physiotherapists. London: Faber & Faber, 1982. ISBN 0 571 18038 8.

Drummond A. Research Methods for Therapists. London: Chapman & Hall, 1996. ISBN 0 412 45950 7.

Ebrahim S. Clinical Epidemiology of Stroke. Oxford: Oxford University Press, 1990. ISBN 0 19 261749 4.

Edwards S. Neurological Physiotherapy: A problem-solving approach. Edinburgh: Churchill Livingstone, 1996. ISBN 0 443 04887 8.

Eggers O. Occupational Therapy in the Treatment of Adult Hemiplegia. Oxford: Heinemann Medical, 1986. ISBN 0 433 08170 8.

Evans J, Wilson B, Emslie H. Selecting, Administering and Interpreting Cognitive Tests. Bury St Edmunds: Thames Valley Test Company, 1996. ISBN 1 874261 06 7.

Greenhalgh T. How to Read a Paper. London: BMJ Publishing Group, 1997. ISBN 0 7279 1139 2.

Grieve J. Neuropsychology for Occupational Therapists, Assessment of Perception and Cognition. Oxford: Blackwell Science, 2000. ISBN 0 632 05067 5.

Hagedorn R. Occupational Therapy: Perspectives and Processes. Edinburgh: Churchill Livingstone, 1995. ISBN 0 443 04978 5.

Hagedorn R. Occupational Therapy: Foundations for Practice. Edinburgh: Churchill Livingstone, 1995. ISBN 0 443 04540 2.

Harrison M. Physiotherapy in Stroke Management. Edinburgh: Churchill Livingstone, 1995. ISBN 0 443 05228 X.

Humphreys GW, Riddoch MJ. To See but Not to See. A Case Study of Visual Agnosia. Hillsdale, NJ: Lawrence Erlbaum Associates, 1987. ISBN 0 86377 065 7.

Jenkins S, Price CJ, Straker L. The Researching Therapist. Edinburgh: Churchill Livingstone, 1998. ISBN 0 443 05761 3.

Laidler P. Stroke Rehabilitation – Structure and Strategy. London: Chapman & Hall, 1994. ISBN 0 412 46950 2.

Langhorne P, Dennis M. Stroke Units: An Evidence Based Approach. London: BMJ Books, 1998. ISBN 0 7279 1211 9.

Lezak MD. Neuropsychological Assessment. Oxford: Oxford University Press, 1995. ISBN 0 19 509031 4.

Lubbock G. Stroke Care, an Interdisciplinary Approach. London: Faber & Faber, 1983. ISBN 0 571 13069 0.

Lynch M, Grisogona V. Stroke and Head Injuries. London: John Murray, 1994. ISBN 0 7195 4697 4.

Miller E. Recovery and Management of Neuropsychological Impairments. Chichester: Wiley, 1985. ISBN 0 471 10532 5.

Miller N. Dyspraxia and its Management. Beckenham: Croom Helm, 1986. ISBN 0 7099 3553 6.

Muir-Giles G, Clark-Wilson J. Brain Injury Rehabilitation: A Neurofunctional Approach, Therapy in practice No. 33. London: Chapman & Hall, 1992. ISBN 156 593 0525.

Mulley G. Practical Management of Stroke. London: Chapman & Hall, 1985. ISBN 0 412 31940 3.

Penso D. Perceptuo-motor Difficulties. London: Chapman & Hall, 1993. ISBN 0 412 39810 9.

Ryerson S, Levit K. Functional Movement Re-education. Edinburgh: Churchill Livingstone, 1997. ISBN 0 443 08913 2.

Sacks O. The Man who Mistook his Wife for a Hat. London: Picador, 1985. ISBN 0 330 29491 1.

Sohlberg M, Mateer C. Introduction in Cognitive Rehabilitation Theory and Practice. New York: Guildford Press, 1989, Ch. 10. ISBN 0898 627 389.

Springer S, Deutsch G. Left Brain, Right Brain. New York: W.H. Freeman, 1993. ISBN 0 7167 2373 5.

Steiner D, Norman G. Health Measurement Scales. Oxford: Oxford University Press, 1995. ISBN 0 19 262670 1.

Stroke Association: Various Leaflets.

Stroke: Epidemiological, Therapeutic and Socio-economic Aspects, RSM Services, No 99. London: Royal Society of Medicine, 1985. ISBN 0 905958 27 6.

Thompson S, Morgan M. Occupational Therapy for Stroke Rehabilitation. London: Chapman & Hall, 1990. ISBN 0 412 33530 1.

Wade DT. Measurement in Neurological Rehabilitation. Oxford: Oxford Medical Publications, 1992. ISBN 0 19 261954 3.

Wade DT. Stroke, Practical Guidelines for General Practice. Oxford: Oxford Medical Publications, 1988. ISBN 0 19 261760 5.

Walsh K. Neuropsychology – A Clinical Approach. Edinburgh: Churchill Livingstone, 1987. ISBN 0 433 03858 9.

Warlow C et al. Stroke: A Practical Guide to Management. Oxford: Blackwell Science, 1997. ISBN 0 86542 874 3.

Zoltan B, Siev E, Freishtat B. The Adult Stroke Patient: A Manual for Evaluation and Treatment of Perceptual and Cognitive Dysfunction. New Jersey: Slack, 1986. ISBN 1 55642 197 4.

Zoltan B. Vision, Perception and Cognition. New Jersey: Slack, 1996. ISBN 1 55642 265 2.

Useful Assessments

Intervention and Effectiveness

- Assessment of Motor and Process Skills (AMPS) (Fisher, 1999)
- Canadian Occupational Performance Measure (COPM) (Law et al., 1991)

Activities of Daily Living

- Australian ADL index (Spencer et al., 1986)
- Barthel ADL Index (Mahoney and Barthel, 1965; Collin et al., 1988)
- Edinburgh Stroke study (Smith, 1979)
- Edmans ADL index (Edmans and Webster, 1997)
- Frenchay activities index (Holbrook and Skilbeck, 1983; Wade et al., 1985)
- Functional Independence Measure (FIM) (Granger et al., 1986)
- Katz ADL index (Katz et al., 1963)
- Kenny self-care assessment scale (Schoening et al., 1965)
- Northwick Park ADL index (Benjamin, 1976)
- Nottingham 10 point ADL scale (Ebrahim et al., 1985)
- Nottingham extended ADL scale (Nouri and Lincoln, 1987)
- Pulses profile (Granger et al., 1979)
- Rivermead ADL assessment (Whiting and Lincoln, 1980; Lincoln and Edmans, 1990)
- Sheikh et al. modified ADL index (Sheikh et al., 1979)

Sensation

- Nottingham Sensory Assessment (Lincoln et al., 1991)
- Rivermead Assessment of Somatosensory Performance (RASP) (Winward et al., 2000)

Attention

- Test of Everyday Attention (TEA) (Robertson et al., 1994)

Cognition

- Middlesex Elderly Assessment of Mental State (MEAMS) (Golding, 1989)

Memory

- Recognition Memory Test (Warrington, 1984)
- Rivermead Behavioural Memory Test (RBMT) (Wilson et al., 1985)
- Salford Objective Recognition Test (SORT) (Burgess et al., 1994)
- Subjective Memory Questionnaire (Bennett-Levy and Powell, 1980)
- Wechsler Memory Scale (Wechsler, 1987)

Reasoning

- Cognitive Estimates (Shallice and Evans, 1978)
- Coloured Progressive Matrices (Raven, 1958)
- Modified Card Sorting Test (Nelson, 1976)
- Word Fluency (from Multilingual Aphasia Examination) (Benton and Hamsher, 1989)

Perception

- Chessington Occupational Therapy Neurological Assessment Battery (COTNAB) (Tyerman et al., 1986)
- Loewenstein Occupational Therapy Cognitive Assessment (LOTCA) (Itzkovich et al., 1993)
- Rey figure copying test (Rey, 1959)
- Rivermead Behavioural Inattention Test (BIT) (Wilson et al., 1987)
- Rivermead Perceptual Assessment Battery (RPAB) (Whiting et al., 1985; Lincoln and Edmans, 1989)
- Visual Object & Spatial Perception Test (VOSP) (Warrington and James, 1991)

Apraxia

- Kertesz Apraxia Test (Kertesz and Ferro, 1984)

Executive Functions

- Behavioural Assessment of the Dysexecutive Syndrome (BADS) (Wilson et al., 1996)
- Hayling and Brixton tests (Burgess and Shallice, 1997)

Anxiety and Depression

- The Hospital Anxiety and Depression scale (Zigmond and Snaith, 1983)
- Wakefield Depression Inventory (Snaith et al., 1971)

- Geriatric Depression Scale (Agrell and Dehlin, 1989)
- General Health Questionnaire (Goldberg and Hiller, 1979)

Driving

- Stroke Drivers Screening Assessment (Nouri and Lincoln, 1994)

Useful Addresses

Chest, Heart and Stroke Scotland
65 North Castle Street
Edinburgh EH2 3LT
Tel: 0131 225 6963

Different Strokes
Sir Walter Scott House
2 Broadway Market
London E8 4QJ
Tel: 020 7249 6645

Health Education Authority
Hamilton House
Mabledon Place
London WC1H 9T
Tel: 020 7222 5300

Medical Disability Society
The Royal College of Physicians
11 St Andrews Place
Regents Park
London NW1 4LE
Tel: 020 7935 1174

NFER-Nelson
Darville House
2 Oxford Road East
Windsor
Berkshire SL4 1DF
Tel: 01753 858 961

The Psychological Corporation Ltd
24–28 Oval Road
London NW1 7DX
Tel: 020 7267 4466

Stroke Association
Stroke House
Whitecross Street
London EC1Y 8JJ
Tel: 020 7566 0300

Thames Valley Test Company Ltd
7–9 The Green
Flempton
Bury St. Edmunds
Suffolk IP28 6EL
Tel: 01284 728 608

Stroke Association Publication List

The following are currently available from the Stroke Association:

Leaflets

S1	Stroke – questions and answers
S2	Learning to speak again
S11	What is TIA?
S15	Epilepsy after stroke
S16	Sex after stroke illness
S17	Carotid endarterectomy
S18	Swallowing difficulties
S23	Central post-stroke pain
S27	Aspirin and stroke
SF1	Introducing the Stroke Association
SF11	High blood pressure?
SF12	Stroke: Know the warning signs
SF14	A hundred years of caring
SW1	Blood pressure and stroke

Booklets

S4	Starting a stroke club/stroke support group
S8	Our games book
S9	Psychological effects of stroke
S13	Stroke and continence
S19	Stroke and wheelchairs
S20	Stroke in younger adults
S22	Driving after stroke
S25	Cognitive problems following stroke
S26	Grandpa's had a stroke
S28	Keeping well after your stroke
S29	After your stroke: a first guide

S30   How to reduce your risk of stroke
S31   Stroke: a carer's guide
S32   Stroke: a guide to your rehabilitation
S33   The reluctant exerciser's guide
SF13   A step-by-step guide to making a will

Books

T1   A Time to Speak
T2   A Stroke in the Family
T8   Puzzle Book
T13   Get Moving

Posters

P16   Stroke: know the warning signs (A4 or A3)
SW2/3 Blood pressure and stroke (A4 or A3)

Other Material

N4   Singalong audio tape and songbook
N5   Word and picture chart
N1   Plastic ID card
Stroke Care – A Matter of Chance. A national survey of stroke services
Stroke Care: Reducing the Burden of Disease
Stroke – Good Practice Resource Pack
Stroke – Resource Pack for Primary Care Groups

Quarterly Magazine

Stroke News

Index